4 x4

Cauliflower   1.84
avacado   1.78
asparagus   1.43
spinach

Keto Diet

90 Days to a New You! The
Ultimate Plan to Lose Over 30
Pounds Without the Gym!

Fitness & Health Fuel

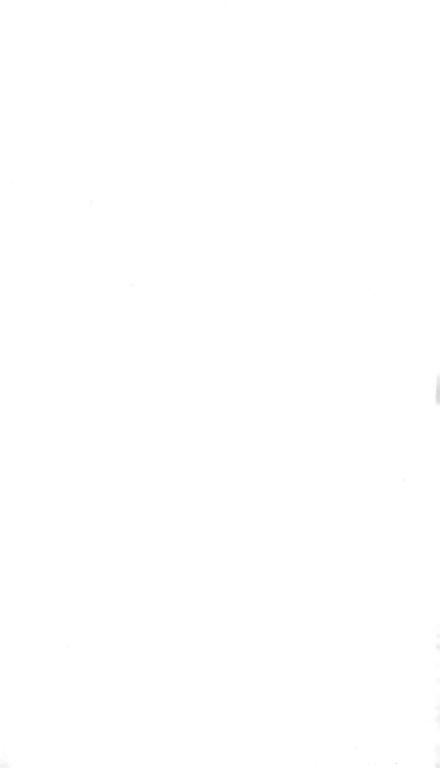

advice. The content of this book has been derived from various sources. Please consult a licensed professional before attempting any techniques outlined in this book.

By reading this document, the reader agrees that under no circumstances are is the author responsible for any losses, direct or indirect, which are incurred as a result of the use of information contained within this document, including, but not limited to, —errors, omissions, or inaccuracies.

WAIT! Sign Up Now And

Get A FREE Bonus!

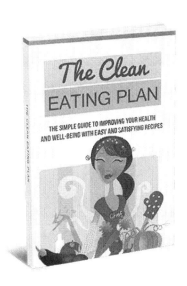

Discover How To Finally Take Control Of Your Diet And Eat Cleaner

- Discover how to eat healthier and cleaner without extra effort

- How your body works and how you can lose weight

- **How to train yourself so that you can eat cleaner forever**

- How to set and achieve your short and long term health goals

- **How to minimize time spent preparing meals**

- And so much more...

https://dibblypublishing.com/fht-bonuses

Contents

Chapter One

An Introduction To The

Keto Diet

Introduction

Recent nutritional research has led to the development of numerous special diets that provide a variety of health benefits. As a result, controlling diseases associated with dieting has been made simpler and more successful. Nonetheless, a lot of people still aren't aware of the existence of such plans.

One such revolutionary diet is the Ketogenic Diet, also referred to as the Keto Diet. The purpose of this book is to teach you, the reader, about the many benefits associated with this unique diet plan.

What is the Keto Diet?

The Keto Diet is an eating plan which focuses on

reducing carbohydrate intake while increasing the intake of fats. This diet recommends eating high-fat foods and adequate protein while keeping carbs low. According to experienced dieticians and nutritionists, the key to keto is making fats the main form of energy in the body.

When you eat foods rich in carbs, the body produces glucose and insulin. Glucose is the easiest molecule for the body to convert and use as energy. Thus, logically, it's the body's preferred energy source. After glucose is consumed and broken down, the liver produces insulin to help with distributing glucose into the bloodstream. Therefore, on a high-carb diet, the body will use glucose as its main source of energy, rather than fat. Fat therefore ends up being stored in the body—not what any dieter wants.

However, lowering the intake of carbs induces the body into a state known as ketosis. During ketosis, the body produces small fuel molecules called ketones. These ketones then serve as an alternative fuel for the body when glucose is in short supply.

Ketones are produced in the liver as a product of the synthesis of fat. The ketones are then transferred throughout the body, including the brain, which requires continuous energy replenishment. Mostly, the energy comes from glucose or ketones.

As mentioned earlier, the Ketogenic Diet involves using fat as the body's sole source of energy. Therefore, the body switches its fuel supply to run entirely on ketones—broken-down fat molecules. Insulin levels are lowered and therefore the fat-burning process spontaneously increases.

Through ketosis, accessing fats in the body and burning them off as energy becomes easy. Though this is a great way to lose weight, it is not the only benefit of ketosis. This book provides many other reasons for why the Keto Diet is so healthy. This book will also discuss a variety of foods to be consumed as well as those to be avoided. Note that you can only reap the full benefits of the Keto Diet if you follow it completely and consistently, rather than sporadically. Remember, this diet is a solution to weight loss troubles and provides many other benefits. Consider it akin to a medical prescription.

History and Origin of the Keto Diet

Even though the Keto Diet has become popular the last two or three decades, it was used in the 1920s as an alternative to non-mainstream fasting which was a successful therapy for epilepsy. Over time, the diet was abandoned due to the introduction of new anticonvulsant therapies.

However, research eventually showed that the

anticonvulsant therapies failed to achieve full seizure control in around 20 to 30 percent of epileptic cases, mainly children. For this reason, the diet was reintroduced as the only known natural method for controlling the condition.

In the ancient world, the role of fasting in managing epilepsy had been studied in detail by Greek physicians and Indian doctors. However, it couldn't be used to fully curb epilepsy, because extended fasting can hurt anyone, especially children. The first modern scientific study to establish the role of fasting in curing epilepsy was conducted in France in 1911. At this time, a drug made up of potassium bromide was being used to treat epilepsy. However, the drug affected brain function, slowing mental processes. This side effect reignited scientists' interest in studying how the Keto Diet could be helpful in controlling epilepsy.

Consequently, twenty epileptic patients were put on a low-calorie, vegetarian food plan that was sparingly combined with fasting. Only two patients showed significant improvements. This was discovered to be because most patients didn't fully follow the required dietary restrictions. The two patients who did improve were shown to have better results on the diet than those treated with potassium bromide.

In the early twentieth century, Bernard McFadden, a nutritionist, popularized the idea of fasting as a means of restoring health. One of his students, Hugh Conklin, started using fasting as a treatment technique for controlling epilepsy. Conklin suggested that epileptic attacks were caused by a toxin secreted in the intestine. He proposed that fasting for 18 to 25 days could lessen the levels of the toxin in the body.

He put some epileptic patients on a diet that involved 95 percent water—the "water diet." As a result, 90 percent of suffering children were cured. Furthermore, 50 percent of adults were fully cured of the disease while the other half showed a huge improvement. Fasting was thus adopted as part of mainstream therapy for epilepsy in 1916.

In 1921, Rollin Woodyatt, an endocrinologist, embarked on research to establish more viable solutions to epilepsy. His findings noted that three water-soluble compounds, acetone, hydroxybutyrate, and acetoacetate were produced by the liver as a result of starvation. Also, he noticed that the three compounds followed a diet rich in fat and low in carbohydrates. As a result of this research, the Mayo Clinic's Russel Wilder called this the "Ketogenic Diet" and used it as a treatment for epilepsy.

More research conducted in the 1960s showed that more ketones are produced by medium-chain triglycerides (MCTs) per unit of energy. This is because ketones are produced and transferred to the liver via the hepatic portal vein as opposed to the lymphatic system.

It is clear that the need for a cure for epilepsy led to the discovery of the Keto Diet. However, we now know that the diet provides a solution for a number of health problems. Nevertheless, many people today use the Keto Diet for weight loss, rather than to combat diseases. Later on in this book, we will discuss keto in the modern world.

Health Benefits of the Keto Diet

What health benefits does the Keto Diet provide? This is one of the most common questions people ask. While other diets have one single benefit—weight loss—the Keto Diet has many health benefits, due to how it changes the body chemistry. The body becomes more efficient when it uses ketones as a fuel source. Below are the key health benefits that come from the Keto Diet.

Enhances Weight Loss

The Keto Diet meal plan has proven to be an efficient method for losing weight. Essentially, the diet uses body fat as a source of energy. This use of fat then leads to weight loss. While on the plan, your insulin levels drop greatly and this turns your body into a fat-burning system. According to various nutritionists, the Keto Diet is a long-term solution for weight loss, offering better results than a low-fat, high-carb diet plan.

How does the actual weight loss process work? When ketosis begins in the body, both blood sugar and insulin levels drop. Fat cells then release the water they retain. This is why most people witness a big drop in weight loss immediately after they start the Keto Diet. After this water loss, the fat cells become small enough to enter the bloodstream and into the liver, where they can be converted to ketones. This process continues as one continues to consistently follow the Keto Diet.

Cancer Prevention and Treatment

Cancer cells are known to survive with glucose as a fuel source. As a result, ketosis has recently become a popular form both of cancer treatment and prevention. Since eating a ketogenic diet deprives cancer cells of glucose, this starves the cancer cells and results in their death.

How, exactly, the Ketogenic Diet is so effective in combating cancer is still not clear. However, preclinical results have displayed safe, significant improvement in a Murine Cancer Model. A study found that ketone supplementation decreased tumor cell viability and extended survival rates in a mouse with cancer.

A study was conducted in 2012 to determine the Keto Diet's actual effect on cancer. The study involved 10 cancer patients who were put on the Keto Diet for 28 days, after exhausting every other cancer treatment option.

Amazingly, the study found that one patient had a partial remission of their cancer, five patients were stabilized, and four continued recuperating. This proves that the Keto Diet causes a huge improvement in treating cancer.

Improving Appetite Control

An amazing thing happens when you eat a low-carb diet: you don't feel hungry often. Additionally, you end any cravings that may cause you to develop bad eating habits.

Most people who adopt the Keto Diet plan are able to engage in intermittent fasting where they only eat during a specific time of the day. This is possible because you will develop the ability to control your appetite.

Better Mental Focus

Medical research has proved that fatty acids have a huge impact on the brain's operations. Specifically, various people have used the Keto Diet to boost their brain performance. The fats ingested on the eating plan are broken down into fatty acids in the digestive system. In turn, this gives the brain the source of fuel it needs to be sharper and more focused, which increases concentration.

According to dieticians, low-carb diets are therapeutic for several brain disorders. This is associated with the usage of ketones as the source of fuel for the brain. Ketones are a reliable and consistent source of fuel which enables one to engage the brain and focus for a longer period of time.

Dissemination of More Energy Within the Body

The body can only store a small amount of glycogen at a time. This makes it necessary to refuel the energy levels in your body from time to time. However, there is a high tendency of the body to store more fats as compared to glycogen. Those fats can be utilized in ketosis, providing a super-self-sufficient source of energy which does not run out easily. On the Keto Diet, the body generates enough energy levels to carry you throughout your day.

Helps Fight Type 2Diabetes

Various studies have shown that following the Keto Diet reduces the chance of type 2 diabetes. Basically, type 2diabetes causes the pancreas to increase insulin production. The Keto Diet removes sugars from the ingredients of every meal. This helps to lower the Hemoglobin A1c levels (the measure which identifies average plasma glucose concentration). As a result, most cases of type 2diabetes are reversed.

Increases Levels of HDL Cholesterol

Don't panic when you hear that the Keto Diet increases the levels of a certain type of cholesterol in the body. Not all cholesterol is bad. Here, we are focusing on healthy HDL cholesterol.

HDL carries cholesterol from the body to the liver, where it is reused or excreted. On the other hand, LDL carries cholesterol from the liver to the rest of the body.

When you follow the Keto Diet, the levels of triglycerides in the body decrease. Simultaneously, HDL levels increase. The triglycerides: HDL ratio is a strong indicator of the possibility of heart disease. The higher it is, the greater your risk of heart disease and vice versa.

Lowering Blood Pressure

High blood pressure is a major indicator for future heart problems. Because the diet leads to a great improvement of triglyceride and cholesterol levels in the body—both linked with arterial buildup—the Keto Diet helps to lower blood pressure.

The low-carb and high-fat Keto Diet results in a rapid increase in HDL and reduction of LDL particle concentration compared to low-fat diets. In turn, this reduces blood pressure better than any other diet. Moreover, effective weight loss, a key result of following this diet, is a major reason for the reduction of blood pressure.

Enhancing the Fight against Metabolic Syndrome

Metabolic syndrome isn't comprised of just one disorder. It is a set of risk factors which combine to significantly raise the risk of heart disease, stroke, and diabetes.

Metabolic syndrome includes the following risk factors.

- High blood pressure

- Low levels of HDL cholesterol

- High blood sugar

- High triglycerides

- Obesity

Metabolic syndrome is becoming a particularly pervasive problem in today's world because more people are suffering from obesity. Researchers believe that metabolic syndrome may soon overtake the use of tobacco as the main cause of heart disease.

Changing one's lifestyle is vital to treating metabolic syndrome. The key element of that lifestyle change is dieting. A diet containing less carbs (the Keto Diet) is an ideal example of a dietary change that has an immense impact on treating, and possibly curing, metabolic syndrome in the long run.

Stable Vision; Less Risk of Cataracts

High blood sugar has a detrimental effect on eyesight. In fact, high blood pressure may increase the risk for cataracts. Lowering blood pressure using the Keto Diet therefore improves eye and vision health.

According to recent research, the majority of people following the Keto Diet have improved their vision. Moreover, they are less likely to develop cataracts than those not on the Keto Diet.

Control of Polycystic Ovary Syndrome (PCOS)

Oftentimes, PCOS occurs as a result of insulin resistance. Insulin resistance disorder is responsible for causing a range of hormonal issues in women, including infertility. Due to the low carbs in the Keto Diet, insulin resistance is tamed. A pilot study has been carried out to establish the significance of the Keto Diet in the regulation of PCOS. The feedback from the study indicated an improvement in body weight, insulin control, and testosterone levels in women. With this management of their PCOS, women could become pregnant.

Overcoming Irritable Bowel Syndrome (IBS)

Irritable bowel syndrome causes chronic diarrhea, stomach discomfort, and bloating among other stomach disorders. People who suffer from IBS are advised to follow a high-fat and low-carb diet—the Keto Diet. At first, increasing fat intake can lead to increased diarrhea. However, the long-term effects of the Keto Diet are soothing to the stomach and end the diarrhea problem.

Numerous studies have indicated that low sugar consumption can assist in tackling IBS symptoms. A particular study found that the Keto Diet reduces abdominal pain, betters bowel movements, and improves quality of life in individuals suffering from IBS

Boosting Endurance

Studies conducted on ketosis paint a clear picture of the relationship between the Keto Diet and endurance. Recent research on fat utilization and performance, dubbed the FASTER study, indicated that people on the Keto Diet have more mitochondria. Furthermore, the same people experience low oxidative stress and a lower lactate load, all of which can lead to lower endurance.

Athletes who adopt the Keto Diet and are more likely to be able to perform at a higher intensity than their counterparts who do not follow the diet. Also, numerous scientific studies have shown that ketones in the blood have a significant positive impact on performance.

Autism Stabilization

Recent research into the potential therapeutic use of the Keto Diet in autism spectrum disorders discovered that the diet is beneficial in dealing with autism. However, more research is needed to determine the success levels of the Keto Diet in fully resolving autism.

One study was done on 30 children suffering from autism. A Keto Diet with 30 percent Medium Chain Triglyceride Oils (MCT oils) was administered for at least six months. Over half of these children with milder autistic behaviors showed the most improvement while the rest displayed mild to moderate improvements.

Epilepsy Treatment

As explained in a prior section of the book, the Keto Diet was first introduced and used in 1921 to treat drug-resistant epilepsy in children. Traditionally, it started as a therapy for children but was adopted to also deal with epilepsy in adults. Since then, a number of studies have been carried out to show how ketosis can help in dealing with epilepsy.

Similar to the stabilization of autism discussed earlier, there is clear evidence of improvement in epilepsy.

Furthermore, using a Keto Diet allows people suffering from epilepsy to take fewer or no anti-epileptic drugs while remaining seizure-free. This can go a long way in reducing the potential side effects of drugs and improving mental performance.

Fighting Cardiovascular Disease

Contrary to the notion of many people, heart problems are not associated with a High-fat Diet. On the other hand, a high carb Diet is highly attributed to some heart complications. This makes a high-fat-low-carb Diet one of the biggest health benefits of the Keto Diet to remember when it comes to heart diseases.

We have looked at the Keto Diet in relation to cholesterol levels. It is prudent to note the different types of cholesterol and their different effects on the body. Conventional information has in the past indicated that we should cut out the intake of meat, eggs, and dairy products. All of this is uninformed thinking since all these ingredients are important constituents of the Keto Diet.

Studies on the Keto Diet have indicated that it has shown enormous results in:

- Reducing total cholesterol levels

- Increasing low-density lipoprotein particles

- Lowering the insulin that activates cholesterol enzymes

In short, the above results lead to reduced risks of developing cardiovascular diseases and complications.

Dealing with Brain Trauma

A number of early studies show that the Keto Diet have a huge positive impact in improving brain trauma. Many experts ascribe the results to the following facts.

- The Keto Diet reduces complications linked to cognitive ability after a trauma

- The Keto Diet lowers the volume of cortical contusion (a type of brain bruise). However, this depends on the age of the patient. Older people may take a longer time to overcome the brain bruise.

- The Keto Diet fastens the healing of epilepsy. This is beneficial since traumatic brain injuries can often lead to epilepsy.

Improved Respiratory Function

The Keto Diet is known to boost anti-inflammatory mechanisms in the body. In turn, this help in improving the respiratory function of the body. For example, the

Keto Diet has proved to be very helpful in dealing with asthma. Additionally, the Keto Diet helps to tackle respiratory failure. Much of it boils down to something known as the respiratory exchange ratio which depends on two factors:

- How much carbon dioxide one produces

- How much oxygen you use

Patients diagnosed with reparatory disorders often have high carbon dioxide levels. The Keto Diet impacts lead to the respiratory exchange ratio. How does this happen? Researchers believe that reducing the glucose stored in the muscles leads to reduced respiratory exchange ratio.

Combating the Alzheimer's Disease

Millions of adults are faced with the devastating development of the Alzheimer's disease each year. Although the disease is chronic, there are potential high chances to reduce major triggers of the Alzheimer's disease when one gets into ketosis.

Ketones improve the combat of the disease by enhancing the function of the mitochondria. The mitochondria are essential components to healthy cell function. Having healthy and powerful body cells leads to maximum protection against amyloid beta – the main plaque component found on the brains of patients with the Alzheimer's disease.

More studies are underway into the additional benefits of the Keto Diet. The advice of nutritionists and dieticians should not be taken for granted. They have vast experience and knowledge which should be a guarantee that their prescription to use the Keto Diet is in line with the solutions to your health problems. The benefits of the Keto Diet are best experienced in the body, rather than just being read about. So, it is time to put it into a test for your health!

Pros and Cons of the Keto Diet

Even as it has many health benefits, the Keto Diet has its pros and cons. The following section extensively discusses these to help you adopt this diet in the safest, most effective way.

Pros

Enhances sugar detoxification

Evidently, the Keto Diet reduces the amounts of sugar in the body. This is because the diet allows only 25 to 35 grams of carbs at every meal. As a result, most people lessen their intake of sugary foods. Controlling sugar intake is a great way to manage diseases like diabetes.

Protein sparing effect

When you ingest an inadequate amount of protein and calories, they're saved for sparing use by other body functions. Ketosis uses ketones rather than glucose. Therefore, protein oxidation will not produce glucose. This is known as the protein sparing effect. It means that the protein will be used in other important bodily functions while fats are used as the body's source of energy.

Lowering insulin levels

If insulin is left unchecked, it can lead to type 2diabetes. The Keto Diet can help people in lowering insulin levels. Meals prepared in line with Keto Diet guidelines greatly reduce the amount of sugar in one's diet. This lessens the production of insulin. A decrease in insulin promotes the release of vital hormones such as growth hormone. Additionally, lowering insulin levels reduces the risks of inflammation in the body.

Lower carb intake

The Keto Diet reduces the intake of carbs during meals. Commonly, simple carbs break down inside the body to produce glucose, a sugary compound that may spike blood sugar, contributing to fatigue. Therefore, eliminating high levels of carbs through the Keto Diet is of paramount importance in controlling body sugar levels.

Burning fats

The Keto Diet improves the body's ability to exploit stored fats as a source of energy for all body functions. Ketosis turns fat into fuel, preventing fat-related problems such as obesity.

Appetite control

Fat consumption helps control appetite by storing sugar elements in the body. Nutritionists suggest that a low level of sugar (glucose) in the body is the basic explanation for why you feel hungry. Since the ketosis process uses fats as a source of energy instead of sugar compounds, glucose levels are not reduced. Due to this, you will usually feel full while on the Keto Diet.

Fats are good for skin and hair

The Keto Diet boosts the levels of healthy fats in the body. In turn, this increases the levels of fatty acids which are important components in promoting healthier hair. Moreover, fats are key contributors to younger-looking skin.

You Feel More Energetic

Often, many people develop an awful feeling when their body sugar levels shoot downwards. Some people describe the feeling as dizziness and it is mostly accompanied by hunger pangs. The best thing with the Keto diet is that you don't have to go through this feeling. In fact, you will feel a lot more energetic and experiences fewer pangs of hunger throughout the day.

Cons

Even though the Keto Diet is mostly known for its many health benefits, it is prudent to acknowledge some of its shortcomings. The cons of the Keto Diet are as follows.

Following the diet may not be easy

Following the Keto Diet requires consistent commitment. We are living in a busy world and this is not always easy. Moreover, the diet dictates that fat be the main ingredient of every meal. This doesn't sound good to many people. For many of us, it's hard to eat fatty food.

Additionally, the Keto Diet requires 70 to 80 percent fat ingredients, 10 percent carbs, and 15 percent protein in a single meal. Thus, ingredients need to be measured accurately and this is the hardest part of the diet for most people.

Increase in acidity levels in the body

Unused ketones in the body may cause ketoacidosis. Ketones are acidic in nature and ketoacidosis is a hyperacidity state in the body. This can cause death.

It may not be a long-term weight loss solution

As much as it's clear that the Keto Diet causes weight loss, it may not be the magic solution people are searching for. People who want to lose more weight are always looking for new methods such as periodic fasting and endurance training.

May cause micronutrient deficiencies

The Keto Diet is very restrictive and, therefore, a lack of various nutrients in the body may lead to micronutrient deficiencies. For instance, the Keto Diet restricts the intake of carbs. To counter this, one needs to take high-quality multivitamin or mineral supplements twice a day. Fiber supplements are also necessary for the health of the digestive system. These additional supplements can be expensive.

Triggers fatigue and brain fog

For the first few weeks after beginning the Keto Diet, you may experience fatigue and brain fog. This is because the body takes time to adjust to the metabolic shift. This is a major shortcoming of the diet. However, this problem is momentary as the body adjusts to the diet within a few weeks.

Altered blood lipid profile

The Keto Diet may result in fluctuations in the amounts of fats in the body. Consequently, this alteration in the blood lipid profile can cause fatal imbalances of cholesterol levels in the body. Reliable statistics indicate that an altered blood lipid profile either rapidly increases or drastically reduces cholesterol levels in a number of individuals.

Elimination of Fiber from the Diet

Though the diet is rich in heart-healthy fats, it is often low on fiber. Notably, many foods that contain sufficient levels of fiber are left out of the Keto diet. Most of the foods that comprise high fiber content include vegetables and are taken in small and recommended amounts. In turn, this reduces fiber which is important in facilitating smoother digestion.

Other side effects such as bad breath, insomnia, and daytime fatigue may occur while one is on the Keto Diet. Additionally, there is the Keto flu which typically occurs for not more than one week on the Keto diet plan. The Keto diet is prevalent among Keto beginners as the body adjusts to using fat as a source of energy. As the body transits into ketosis, one may experience symptoms like nausea, dizziness, achy muscles, and irritable mood. Once the Keto flu is over, you may feel more energized and alert.

It is imperative to note that the benefits of the Keto diet offset the shortcomings. However, it is also important to take care when you are switching to the diet. Get advice from a nutritionist specialist before making the decision to start the Keto Diet. Be ready to counter the cons of the diet. Ultimately, the health benefits are incomparable to any other diet.

Is the Keto Diet for you?

Maybe. Even as the Keto Diet has shown promising results for cancer, weight loss, and other health issues, many people are not ready to cut down carbs in their meals. Most people say that it is hard to follow the diet for an extended period. Moreover, it is questionable whether the diet is a safe long-term solution to numerous health complications.

There are a number of factors that determine whether or not the Keto Diet is suitable for a person. Lifestyle is one of them. The activities you engage in have a huge influence on whether or not you should follow the Keto Diet. This is because various activity levels require a different type of nutrition. For example, a person who engages in regular intense exercise needs a diet rich in carbs. For this reason, it is wise to fully understand the kinds of activities you engage in on a daily basis before choosing a diet.

Anyone looking to experience any of the health benefits listed in the previous section should try the Keto Diet. However, beginning to use the Keto Diet should not be solely a personal decision. It should also include the advice of a nutritionist, dietician, or your personal doctor. Various tests can be carried out on you to ensure that your body will not negatively react to the Keto Diet. Do not prescribe the Keto Diet to yourself! Follow a medical professionals' advice.

There are several side effects which may emerge as a result of using the diet. Those side effects may be severe if the diet is adopted without the supervision or guidance of a specialist. Some moderate side effects may include bad breath, insomnia, and daytime fatigue. In addition, more complicated side effects may be hyperacidity, acne, and the keto flu, among others. To avoid such problems, make sure you don't just pick up a Keto Diet guide and jump in. Get medical advice first!

Who should not begin a ketogenic diet?

The caution about the Keto Diet's cons should not dissuade you from trying the diet. Nonetheless, there are three groups of people who cannot be advised to begin the Keto Diet. These are:

- Women who are breastfeeding

- People taking medication for high blood pressure

- People taking medication for diabetes

Why it is not advisable for breastfeeding women to begin the Keto Diet

Eating a low-carb diet might be helpful in losing excess pregnancy weight. However, a low-carb diet while breastfeeding may have a potentially dangerous effect on your body. Therefore, you need to choose a diet with a moderately higher level of carbs. For example, you can follow a diet containing at least 50 grams of carbs per day.

How does the Keto Diet specifically affect breastfeeding? Here is a precise explanation.

In normal situations, any woman's body can handle carbs from time to time. Conversely, a large percentage of sugar from a woman's body is lost through milk when breastfeeding. In fact, a breastfeeding woman loses between 30 and 50 grams of sugar per day. Not eating more carbs to help in the replacement of those lost sugars can cause ketoacidosis, a rare, fatal condition. This is a disorder that causes massive dehydration and an abnormal buildup of acids in the body. It also causes altered breathing and type 1 diabetes.

You can overcome ketoacidosis by getting enough nutrients while breastfeeding. Monitor your sugar levels by eating enough carbs. The recommended amount of sugar intake is at least 50 grams per day. One way to ensure that you get enough amount of sugar is by eating three large fruits per day. For example, you can choose to eat three mangos, apples, or any other fruit that you love.

Why it is not advisable for people on medication for high blood pressure to follow the Keto Diet

The Keto Diet is known as a suitable method for controlling high blood pressure. Under the Keto Diet, countless people have been able to lower their blood pressure. However, it is not advisable to combine the Keto Diet with medication for high blood pressure.

What is the danger?

High blood pressure begins to normalize when a patient starts taking medication as prescribed by a physician. However, putting the body on a low-carb diet may inhibit the medication's effects and even cause low blood pressure problems.

Why it is not advisable for people taking medication for diabetes to follow the Keto Diet

Do you have diabetes and use medication like insulin? It is true that the Keto Diet can be effective in controlling diabetes. Nevertheless, you will need to have a clear understanding of the effects of adopting the Keto Diet while you are on diabetes medication. Consuming a low-carb diet can result in a reduction of insulin doses. The Keto Diet lowers the carbs that raise your blood sugar and therefore your medication becomes less important. Some people continue taking the same insulin doses while on the Keto Diet, oblivious to the hidden risks.

Doctors point out the fact that combining medication for diabetes with the Keto Diet might result in hypoglycemia, a situation where the body develops low sugar symptoms. Having the condition is the same as having high sugar levels—the health risks involved are similar. Before adopting the Keto Diet, ensure you test your sugar level regularly. This will help you lower your insulin dosage. A physician *must* be involved in every stage of this endeavor.

Patients suffering from Noninsulin-Dependent Diabetes Mellitus

There is a popular belief that diets rich in carbohydrates causes an increase in risks that lead to the development of Noninsulin-Dependent Diabetes. However, the opposite is true. An increased intake of carbohydrates lowers the risk of developing the complication. Doctors suggest that diets with high amounts of carbs improve the body's sensitivity to insulin. Therefore, patients with Noninsulin-Dependent Diabetes should switch to a high-carb-low-fat diet for effective combating of the disease. This is a clear indication that such patients should forfeit the Keto diet until this type of diabetes is completely curtailed. In addition, the high carb-low fat diet in patients with Noninsulin-Dependent Diabetes reduces the risks of having heart disease which is a major cause of death among people diabetes.

Cholesterol Concerns and Other Concerns About the Keto Diet

Often, people wonder whether the Keto Diet increases cholesterol levels in the body. This section of this book aims to explore that subject. Let us first answer the most common question—what is cholesterol and why do we need it?

Cholesterol is a waxy, fat-like substance that comes from fats. It is very important in maintaining the integrity of body cells. In the body, cholesterol is used to produce hormones such as testosterone, estrogen, and vitamin D. It is also needed for the production of bile acids, which are vital for effective digestion of fats.

The liver and intestines are among the organs that are known to produce most of the cholesterol found in the body. Typically, 75 percent of the body's cholesterol is produced endogenously while the rest is ingested from natural or external sources. Natural sources of cholesterol include meat, cheese, butter, and eggs. A small amount of these items can contain a lot of cholesterol. This means that excessive consumption can lead to high cholesterol levels that may be unnecessary in the body.

Does the Keto Diet raise cholesterol levels in the body?

Even though the Keto Diet is based on high-fat intake, we cannot say that it causes an increase in cholesterol in the body.

Cholesterol levels vary from one person to another, regardless of whether or not they are keto dieters. However, many studies have indicated that one in 10 keto dieters can experience a rise in cholesterol levels. Nevertheless, the resulting amount of cholesterol may not cause imminent danger to the body.

A few years ago, research was carried out to prove the relationship between cholesterol levels and the Keto Diet. The research involved 140 children suffering from epilepsy. It was noted that cholesterol levels had increased by 60 percent among the children after six months on the Keto Diet.

After the epileptic children consistently followed the diet, the results were different. The cholesterol levels diminished. As a result, it was concluded that the long-term effect of the Keto Diet on cholesterol levels is a reduction, rather than an increase.

Another study was conducted on the long-term effects of the Keto Diet in obese patients. The researchers were fascinated to find out cholesterol levels were reduced within 24 weeks on the Keto Diet. In fact, the diet lowered total cholesterol levels, increased HDL (good) cholesterol, and trimmed triglyceride levels in the obese patients.

Types of cholesterol

Cholesterol is commonly transported in the body by molecules composed of proteins called lipoproteins. The types of cholesterol vary in density. The most researched types, because of their impact on the body, are Low-Density Lipoproteins (LDL) and High-Density Lipoproteins (HDL). They are also frequently used as clinical indicators for different health conditions.

What is HDL cholesterol?

HDL cholesterol is generally called good cholesterol. This is because it can be transported back to the liver for recycling or to be destroyed. Due to this, HDL cholesterol does not accumulate and clog arteries, so it doesn't have a negative effect on cardiovascular health. In addition, HDL cholesterol is associated with anti-inflammatory benefits. HDL reduces inflammatory activity by regulating immune system cells called macrophages.

What is LDL cholesterol?

LDL transports cholesterol produced by the liver and other organs throughout the body. LDL molecules move slowly through the bloodstream and may become oxidized. Once oxidized, LDL may easily burrow into the walls of the arteries and hamper cardiovascular functions. In turn, this triggers an inflammatory response in which the red blood cells rush to "eat up" the LDL molecules.

Increased levels of LDL cholesterol are associated with an increased risk of cardiovascular disease. Moreover, a recent study has shown a strong correlation between LDL cholesterol and an increase in heart-related disorders. The tendency of LDL cholesterol to cause health complications is the reason why it is called bad cholesterol.

LDL particles and heart disease

Experts believe that LDL cholesterol molecules are responsible for causing heart disease. When LDL molecules are oxidized in the bloodstream, they enter the arterial wall and begin atherosclerosis—artery wall clogging. This makes the artery thicker on the inside, reducing its normal capacity. In turn, this makes the heart struggle to pump blood through the thickened arteries.

Generally, the heart will start straining to pump blood.

In most cases, the heart muscles begin to wear out. Your heart cannot pump blood to body organs as usual. In the long run, the heart muscles die out and you are no more.

Does saturated fat increase LDL cholesterol?

Yes! Saturated fats have been proven to raise LDL cholesterol levels. Saturated fats include acidic compounds such as palmitic, myristic, and lauric acid which make up a large portion of milk fat. On the other hand, high-fat dairy produce has been shown to have several cardioprotective benefits.

Therefore, even as avoiding all dairy fat may lower LDL cholesterol, it may not be a good thing for your health. Lowering saturated fat intake by replacing it with unsaturated fats will lower total LDL cholesterol and decrease the risk of cardiovascular and heart diseases. LDL cholesterol response to the intake of saturated fats may vary from one person to another. Some people experience an increase while others witness a reduction or no change at all.

Chapter Two

Ketosis And Weight Loss

Losing Weight With the Keto Diet

The Keto Diet is associated with helping people lose weight and shed body fat. In fact, a number of studies suggest that the Keto Diet is more effective than conventional diets and other methods of weight loss. The Keto Diet is more reliable in providing weight loss solutions because it prescribes highly satiating whole foods while eliminating high levels of carbs. Such a diet makes one feel full. Therefore, one eats fewer calories and loses weight.

It is wise to be persistent and consistent while on the Keto Diet. Nutritionists recommend that people approach the Keto Diet with an open mind. Don't have any preconceived notions and instead be ready to experience the benefits yourself. Furthermore, make it a long-term diet. Don't give up within the first few days because you feel some side effects. Rather, take your time, consult your nutritionist, and work with him or her to address the issues that may be making you feel uncomfortable.

How Fast Will You Lose Weight With the Keto Diet?

This is a common question. Well, here is the best answer!

Once you go through the first week of the Keto Diet, your body is already in ketosis. This means that you will soon start to shed a large amount of body fat. The weight loss at this stage is around one to two pounds a week, mostly from body fat.

As you get closer to your target weight, it's advisable to get the advice of a specialist in determining whether or not to stay on the Keto Diet. Continuing the Keto Diet for weight loss even after attaining one's target weight can be fatal.

The relationship between ketosis and weight loss

Lowering your carb intake for a couple of days as you begin the Keto Diet triggers the ketosis process. As indicated earlier, this process turns fat compounds into ketones. Ketones act as an alternative fuel source which has uncountable benefits for the brain and the nervous system.

Apart from creating a source of fuel for the body, ketosis promotes weight loss. Once the body enters ketosis, a keto dieter starts consuming fewer calories, resulting in more weight loss.

The other reason why the Keto Diet is attributed to effective weight loss is that ketones have a mild diuretic effect, meaning they cause water loss. The mild diuretic effect sucks water from all body parts and "shrinks" the body. People should know that the rapid weight loss is not only from the loss of fats but also due to water loss.

Following are some points you need to consider when you intend to use the keto diet for weight loss.

The weight loss process may not be consistent—there are weeks where you may not notice any weight loss. This doesn't mean that the Keto Diet is ineffective. You should continue on the diet to ensure your body adjusts as necessary in order to enter maximum ketosis. Be patient and do not be discouraged.

Eat the right amount of proteins—too much protein can cause an increase in insulin levels. In turn, this reduces ketone levels. Failure to consume enough protein may cause the ketosis process to burn muscle mass rather than body fat. A standard protein intake should range from 0.6g to 1g per lean pound of body mass.

Supplement the Keto Diet with MTCs. Medium Chain Triglycerides (MTCs) are special types of saturated fats that undergo ketosis to form ketones. MTCs increase satiety (fullness) and therefore reduce food intake. Simultaneously, they enhance cognitive performance and energy levels in the body. This means that MTCs are perfect weight loss supplements for keto dieters.

Take calorie deficit breaks (diet breaks) every two weeks. Caloric deficit breaks result in more weight loss. This method of dieting helps to keep the body from slowing down, allowing you to burn more calories while in a calorie deficit break.

Few people who have been reported to overdo the Keto Diet for weight loss purposes may experience more complications than benefits. Losing weight above the necessary levels leads to a low Body Mass Index (BMI). Note that when you have a low BMI, you are deemed to be somewhat underweight. This may amount to a number of negative health issues emanating from a comprised immune system. The worse scenario associated with low BMI in women is an increased risk of miscarriage. According to a recent study, women who may lose exceedingly more weight than the recommended levels are 72 percent more likely to experience a miscarriage. Take care and don't become a victim of excess weight lose!

Macros and Tracking

"Macros" is short for macronutrients. Macros are the energy-giving components of food that fuel the body. The three main macros relatable to the Keto Diet include carbohydrates (carbs), proteins, and fats. Most calories in the body come from these macros. It is important to know the composition of macros in the Keto Diet to enhance the diet's health benefits.

All three macros have different effects on ketosis depending on their digestion. They have a consequent effect on the levels of blood glucose and hormones.

Typically, fats are 90 percent ketogenic and 10 percent anti-ketogenic. This is due to small amounts of glucose released during the conversion of triglycerides. On the other hand, proteins are 45 percent ketogenic and 55 percent anti-ketogenic. This is because proteins are converted to both glucose and insulin. In turn, the insulin levels rise to over half of the consumed protein and become converted into glucose. Additionally, carbs are 100 percent anti-ketogenic. They contain high levels of glucose and insulin in the blood.

Proteins and carbohydrates influence how our bodies transition into ketosis. The most important thing is to understand how these nutrients are utilized as a form of energy after we ingest macronutrients.

Therefore, it is imperative to comprehend how each of the macros impacts the body in the transition, in order to maximize ketosis. The following are explanations on how the macros are utilized for energy.

Proteins

Proteins are vital nutrients in the Keto Diet. However, they are only included in the diet because it is wise and healthy to have a balanced diet at all times. Eating more than the recommended amounts of proteins will derail ketosis. As indicated earlier, massive amounts of proteins lead to a high production of glucose in the body. This is against the aim of the Keto Diet—to use fats as the body's main source of energy, as opposed to glucose.

Therefore, proteins are not to be eaten in large quantities as part of the Keto Diet. Proteins are only 45 percent ketogenic. This means that eating more proteins will slow ketosis.

Fats

The Keto Diet is known as a high-fat diet. Fat intake determines how successful the Keto Diet becomes to our bodies. Fats are 90 percent ketogenic and the body can scoop significant amounts from a fat intake. Some fat components, such as glycerol from triglycerides, may be changed into glucose. Nevertheless, this is a negligible amount of glucose produced and cannot lower ketosis.

Mostly, fats are consumed during the day and not specifically in one meal. This causes the body to use the glucose produced without affecting ketosis. Unhealthy fats should be avoided since they may have a fatal impact on ketosis, slowing down the absorption of proteins needed in the body.

Carbs

These are the most restricted nutrients in the Keto Diet as they have the biggest negative impact on ketosis. Carbs are the biggest source of blood sugars, which disrupt ketosis. The general rule is that one should not consume more than 30 grams of carbs in a keto meal.

When carbs are processed in the digestive system, they are converted into a considerable amount of glucose. The sugars enter the bloodstream, where they are either burned for energy or stored as glycogen. Regular consumption of excess carbs may lead to sugar imbalance-related diseases such as diabetes.

Calories in the Keto Diet

It is important to regulate the amounts of calories you eat while on the Keto Diet as they can cause a negative impact on ketosis. A person's caloric requirements may be determined by the level of activities engaged in on a normal day. Maintaining or losing weight requires serious calorie control.

Tracking Your Macros

Generally, tracking macros means monitoring the levels of macronutrients consumed. It is easier to track your macros while on the Keto Diet.

Tracking your macros is important, especially when:

- You are a beginner in the Keto Diet. Entering ketosis requires lightly different levels of macros. It is important to monitor your intake in order to obtain the recommended levels of ketosis.

- You are following the Keto Diet for weight loss. Obviously, not consuming appropriately balanced macros will affect a person's weight loss.

Do not obsess about tracking the right amounts of macros. That can cause stress, which is not healthy for ketosis. Instead, try to make the tracking process easier and more efficient by finding the balance of the right amounts of carbs, protein, and fats to reach full ketosis. Furthermore, you can do the following to track your macros:

- Identify your health goals – people on the Keto Diet have different objectives. For example, some do the diet to lose weight, build muscle, need to be able to pinpoint the main goal. This way, you will have a defined level of macros to adhere to.

- Determine the amounts of macros you eat. You can do this from macro amount values suggested by a nutritionist or from a certified online macro calculator.

- Calculate the macros in any food you want to eat, following the nutritional label on most packaged foods. The information includes different ingredients and their corresponding macro amounts.

- Create a meal plan based on ketogenic foods. The meal plan will help to ensure that you eat foods rich in the macros specifically required by ketosis.

Importance of Tracing Macros

Tracking macros in every diet is vital in making the Keto successful. Why is it important to track macros? Keto dieters who count macros make up about 80 percent of their meals from healthy foods listed in the Keto diet food list. Below are the main benefits of keeping a track of the macros you should take in every Keto meal.

You gain more knowledge about food

While tracking macro, it will surprise you to know what nutritional value some foods contain. Tracking macros enlighten dieters to understand the kind of food with high or low levels of each macro. This way, you even gain more knowledge on how to make better and healthy food choices.

One is more likely to stick to the Keto diet

Most Keto diet beginners break their dieting routine sooner than expected because they feel too restricted. Tracking macros can make room for food substitutes which makes the diet plan more interesting. For instance, one can take some pieces of chocolate, some ice cream among other edibles without ruining the Keto diet plan.

You do not have to fear eating out

While on the Keto diet, it is obvious that one may be restricted to the type of foods to eat. However, tracing macros will change the way you alter the diet plan adverse negative effects. You can still eat out with friends and remain within the confines of the Keto diet. Conduct enough research and eat out in restaurants which offer nutritional information on their menu.

Meal preparation does not take much time

Conventional dietary measures suggest that preparation of meals should take more time, especially while sorting out ingredients for a particular diet. With the Keto diet, tracking of macros will definitely reduce the meal prep time since there is a wide variety of nutritious food. Therefore, your time in the kitchen choosing what to and not to cook will reduce.

How to Enter Ketosis

While on the Keto Diet, the first few days will take you into ketosis. How will you know you are in ketosis? There are a few things that increase your level of ketosis. Following are the key things that get you into ketosis:

- Reduce protein intake – While on the Keto Diet, it is prudent to stick to the levels of proteins indicated by your daily plan. Otherwise, the diet will not be effective because excess proteins reduce ketosis. Recall that proteins are converted to glucose in the body and that, in turn, curtails the ketosis process. If possible, consume less than 1 gram of protein per day per kg of body weight. This means that you can consume around 60 grams of proteins if you weigh 60kgs. It is important to note that consuming more proteins than needed stops the ketosis process. Always take note of the nutritional information to ensure you eat the right amounts of protein.

- Restricting intake of carbs –It is prudent to reduce carbs to a digestible amount. For example, 20 grams or less per day would be an ideal amount. However, fiber intake does not have to be reduced and is important to help keep the digestive system healthy. When the level of carbs is restricted, you enter ketosis more swiftly and efficiently.

- Avoid snacking – You can skip either the 10:00 a.m. or 4:00 p.m. snack if you are not feeling hungry. Eating more than needed slows the ketosis process and slows down weight loss. Ideally, snacks are meant for the moments you feel extremely hungry.

- Adopt some exercises – Combining exercise with a low-carb diet can go a long way in enhancing ketone levels in the body. This increases the rate of weight loss. However, it should be crystal clear that exercising does not in any way lead to ketosis. It only helps to raise the rate of ketosis by facilitating burning more fats in the body.

- Try intermittent fasting – This involves skipping meals, especially when you are not feeling hungry. Periodic fasting can prove very helpful at boosting ketone levels. This accelerates weight loss and also assists in reversing type 2 diabetes.

- Eat sufficient fat – The ketosis process is fueled by fats. Thus, the Keto Diet requires more fats. Lowering your fat consumption will negatively impact ketosis. Consume the recommended amount of fats to aid the ketosis process. Otherwise, your body will burn muscle for energy instead of fat.

- Get enough sleep – Most people sleep for no less than seven hours per night, which qualifies as enough sleep. Getting enough sleep keeps stress under control. Stress is one of the factors that tends to slow the ketosis process. This is because sleep deprivation and an increase of stress hormones in the body raise blood sugar levels. In turn, this slows the ketosis process and weight loss.

How to Know Whether or Not You Are in Ketosis

The importance of ketosis is already clear. How do you know if you are in ketosis? Well, there are a few symptoms that indicate that the ketosis process has begun. Furthermore, it is possible to measure ketosis by testing by testing urine, blood, or breath samples.

First, let's look at the symptoms that show the start of ketosis.

- Dry mouth and increased thirst – A dry mouth is a result of not consuming fluids and electrolytes, like salt. Sometimes a dry mouth can taste metallic from time to time. To solve the problem, drink enough water throughout the day. The ideal amount is eight glasses of water per day. Moreover, one or two cups of bullion per day will also be helpful.

- Increased urination – Within the first few days of the ketosis process, you may need to go to the bathroom more often. Actually, this is the main reason for increased thirst as most of the water in the body is lost through urination.

- Keto breath – One can develop the Keto breath within a couple of days of adopting the Keto diet. It is caused when acetone ketones escape via breathing. Keto breath makes smells fruity or similar to nail polish remover. Sweat can also have the same odor. However, the smell is temporary and does not persist for more than three weeks.

- Reduced hunger – Within the first few days of ketosis, many keto dieters experience a noticeable reduction in hunger. This is attributed to the body's ability to utilize stored fats as a source of energy. Due to this, people are less hungry. At times, reduced hunger lead to intermittent fasting which speeds up weight loss.

- Increased energy – Many people report having increased energy levels after starting the Keto diet. This is a clear indication of the beginning of ketosis.

How to Track Ketone Levels

Tracking ketone levels can be done in three ways. However, these methods all come with pros and cons.

1. Urine trips

2. Breath ketone analyzers

3. Blood ketone meter

Let's look at each method, one at a time.

Urine strips

A ketone compound called acetoacetate may end up in urine, allow for ketone levels to be measured using urine as a specimen. This is the most recommended ketone test for beginners. When testing using this method, dip the strip in a small amount of urine. There will be a change of color on the strip within 15 seconds. A high ketone presence is indicated by a dark purple color on the testing strip.

Pro:

- Urine strips are readily available in most pharmacies

Cons:

- The results depend on how much fluid one drinks.

- Strips do not provide a precise ketone level. (i.e., a specific number)

- As one becomes keto-adapted and remains in ketosis, the body may start reabsorbing ketones from urine. This makes the urine strips unreliable.

Breath Ketone Analyzers

Breath ketone analyzers are small gadgets with which you can measure ketone levels through breath. According to a recent market analysis, breath ketone analyzers are by far much expensive than urine strips. However, the devices are reusable for several other measurements.

These gadgets do not provide a specific ketone level. Instead, they provide a general color code for various ketone levels.

Pros:

- The devices are reusable.

- Breath ketone analyzers are simple test tools that can be used without a manual.

Cons:

- Breath ketone analyzers do not correlate with blood ketones, only acetones which are in the breath within the first few days of being on the Keto Diet.

- They are not accurate and can be misleading on the ketone levels in the blood.

- The gadgets are expensive.

Blood Ketone Meters

Blood ketone meters are the best tools for obtaining an accurate measurement of ketones in the blood. When testing ketone levels with a meter, you just need a small amount of blood which can be obtained by pricking your finger.

Pros:

- Breath ketone analyzers provide an exact number of ketones in the body.

- They are reliable.

Cons:

- The gadgets are extremely expensive.

- If you are unable to purchase a meter, one test at a dispensary costs at least $2. This is expensive if you have to run regular tests as you track your ketone levels.

- It involves pricking your finger for a drop of blood. This may be painful.

What to Expect When You Go Keto

Many people are unaware of what to expect after beginning the Keto Diet. Below is a summary of the major results that everyone can expect after starting the Keto Diet.

Weight loss

This is the biggest reason people start the Keto Diet. Research has shown that the Keto Diet plays an important role in maintaining or shedding weight. The slimming effects of the diet happen for multiple reasons.

- Lower sugar consumption has overall health benefits

- Low carbohydrate consumption leads to additional burned calories

- Ketosis results in body fat being burned, which leads to weight loss

Energy Boost

People who do the Keto Diet experience high, stable energy levels. Due to ketosis, the body's energy levels are continuously replenished. However, beginners experience low energy as the body switches over to ketosis. This should not be cause for alarm as it is a temporary state while the body adjusts.

Anti-inflammatory

Inflammation is a common disorder affecting many people. It is a leading cause of cancer, arthritis, and heart disease, among other chronic health conditions.

According to various studies, sugar is a major cause of inflammation. Since the Keto Diet encourages a lower sugar intake, inflammation will lessen. Consuming plenty of healthy fats, such as omega-3 from fish, also lowers inflammation.

The anti-inflammatory benefit provided by the Keto Diet may also be caused by burning more ketones. This causes the body to produce fewer reactive oxygen species which cause inflammation in the body.

Longevity

The Keto Diet enhances your lifespan. Yes! The Keto Diet helps you live longer and has an anti-aging effect. A study was conducted to determine the cause of heart-related diseases. Surprisingly, a low-carb diet can potentially reduce the risk of the heart disease. Also, saturated fats are less likely to cause a stroke.

According to nutritionists and psychologists, lowering oxidative stress is a great way of improving lifespan. The decrease in oxidative stress is caused by a corresponding reduction of insulin in the body. Even as the Keto Diet reduces insulin levels in the body, it plays a role in the reduction of oxidative stress. Due to this, experts suggest that the overall effect of the reduction of stress increases a person's lifespan. Nutritionists are continuing to research exactly how the Keto Diet slows down aging.

It is worthwhile noting that some people can use the Keto Diet for other health benefits, elaborated upon elsewhere in this book. You can review the benefits, start the Keto Diet, and expect to address the health issues you have.

The Power of Fasting and Ketosis

When dieticians talk about fasting in the context of the Keto Diet, they refer to intermittent fasting. This is when you eat only at specific times and avoid food even when you feel hungry before those scheduled times. People find fasting hard to cope with but it can effectively assist ketosis. Before you get used to fasting, it is advisable to eat a snack before the indicated mealtime.

Fasting by itself is a method and not a diet. Fasting aims at changing our lifestyle and does not have anything to do with what we eat. It is about *when* to eat. Let's take a closer look at intermittent fasting and consider how to apply this method to the Keto Diet.

What is intermittent fasting?

Intermittent fasting involves scheduled eating. Usually, the most suitable time to practice intermittent fasting is between 6-8 hours during the day. Notably, intermittent fasting does not in any way involve a specific diet. It is just a dieting pattern. For example, it may mean skipping breakfast and eating later in the day, around 12:00 to 8:00 p.m.

Other people eat a "heavy" breakfast and eat small meals throughout the day. This may also be a kind of intermittent fasting. Fasting is not new to us. It started a long time ago as a religious endeavor. Additionally, our ancestors went through fasting periods caused by lack of food. Eventually, it was determined to have dietary benefits.

Types of intermittent fasting

There are various types of intermittent fasting that you may engage in:

Eating within a daily window

This type of intermittent fasting entails eating within a specified period of time. For example, you might only plan to eat between 11:00 a.m. and 7:00 p.m. each day. This gives your body ample time for its required caloric intake. However, some people may shorten the daily window to four or six hours within a day.

Fat fast plus intermittent fasting

Fast fasting is abstaining from eating fats for an extended period of time. It is popular in helping to break weight loss plateaus. Fat fasting, combined with intermittent fasting, involves eating fats but only during a certain period of time.

Skipping meals

This is the most prevalent fasting method among many

people. It is a good method for easing into fasting. For example, you can skip breakfast for three days in a week and skip dinner for another three days.

Alternating fasting

Typically, this type of intermittent fasting involves scheduling fasting for a specified number of days and eating during the remaining days. For example, you would plan to fast on weekends and eat for the five days remaining in the week.

Any type of intermittent fasting should be based on the guidance of a dietician. This is mainly because there are a few factors that need to be considered before fasting. For example, your health is key to determining whether or not you should try fasting. You may be taking medication that requires you to eat a lot of food.

The relationship between ketosis and fasting

Fasting provides vital support to the process of ketosis. This is because, as you limit food intake, you cut down on the intake of glucose. Your body starts to look for another source of energy. Ultimately, the only available source of energy is the fat in your body. The fat starts to be processed to produce energy for the body. Burning fat to produce energy is the whole process of ketosis. However, you can still enter ketosis without fasting.

Benefits of intermittent fasting while on keto

There are numerous advantages of fasting while on the Keto Diet.

- You enter ketosis faster – Fasting is effective in helping you to deplete glycogen stores more quickly. Additionally, you also avoid consuming carbs when fasting and this helps you enter ketosis more quickly.

- You drop weight faster – People on the Keto Diet for weight loss may find it helpful to combine fasting and the Keto Diet. Fasting leads you to lose more weight. Not only does your body starts burning body fat faster, you are also not likely to eat much during fasting. This causes faster weight loss.

- Caloric restriction – Intermittent fasting is usually compared to caloric restriction but they are not the same. Intermittent fasting provides a long-term solution to calorie control. Moreover, fasting helps you maintain proper, monitored nutrition and a measured caloric intake, which is vital in promoting weight loss.

- Increased mental clarity – Fasting and ketosis cause the brain to use ketones as its source of energy. Most keto dieters experience a boost in mental clarity and less brain fog.

- You spend less and cook infrequently – Preparing keto meals may cost more compared to normal meals. While skipping meals, you save yourself the hassle of spending money and spending time in the kitchen. Moreover, fasting does away with the worry that comes when keto dieters travel to an area are where keto ingredients are not available.

Combining fasting and the Keto Diet

Combining fasting with the Keto Diet may be a great way to make the ketosis process effective. However, there are a few things you need to keep in mind.

Make sure you are adhering to your macros. Tracking your macros is important to ensure that you consume sufficient amounts. It is also good to stick to sufficient levels of calories during meals.

Note that fasting alone cannot be of any health benefit. Combining fasting with keto meals, enough sleep, and reduction of stress is healthier.

Fasting helps you adapt to the Keto Diet faster. Even if continuous fasting is hard for you, try fasting for a day or two before starting the Keto Diet. Naturally, you will be hungry and craving any type of meal that comes your way. Therefore, eating a keto meal will be easier than when you were on another diet.

Start slow. Some people find it easy to jump right into any dietary change. However, begin the Keto Diet gradually if you are a person that does not easily adapt to dietary changes. Start by substituting regular snacks with keto snacks and then move on to replacing main meals. This gradual introduction to the Keto Diet is good because it does not cause instant changes to the body's metabolism.

Chapter Three

Keto Food List

List of What You Can and Cannot Eat

Do you want to start the Keto Diet but don't know what and what not to eat? It may be challenging to follow a healthy low-carb diet, especially as a beginner. Don't worry. The following provides a comprehensive list of foods you should and should not be eating while following the Keto Diet.

The majority of meals you eat while on the Keto Diet should be made from the complete grocery list included in this book. If mixed, as per the guidelines of the Keto Diet, most of the listed keto ingredients make delicious foods. Don't forget that keto meals should be precisely prepared in order to ensure macros are tracked. Unless this is done, one cannot benefit from the Keto Diet.

In this section, we'll categorize keto foods into three groups: foods to eat freely, foods to eat moderately, and foods to avoid. We'll look at every group at length.

FOODS TO EAT FREELY

Healthy Fats

Fats are the most vital part of a ketogenic recipe. Fat is what supplies energy and prevents hunger, weakness, and fatigue. Therefore, keto meals should have sufficient amounts of healthy fats. Here are the categories of healthy fats you should consume on the Keto Diet.

- Saturated fats such as lard, tallow, chicken fat, duck fat, goose fat, ghee, butter, coconut oil, and MCT oil

- Monounsaturated fats such as avocado oil, macadamia oil, and olive oil

- Polyunsaturated fats including omega-3 fatty acids, especially from animal sources like fatty fish and seafood

Non-Starchy Vegetables

- Spinach, lettuce, chives, endive, radicchio, among others

- Some cruciferous vegetables like kales, kohlrabi, radishes

- Celery stalk, asparagus, cucumber, summer

squash, bamboo shoots

Meats

- Grass-fed beef, lamb, goat, venison (red meat)

- Camel meat

- Wild-caught fish and seafood, pastured pork and poultry, pastured eggs

- Offal from grass-fed animals such as liver, heart, kidneys, and other organ meats

- *Avoid farmed fish*

- *Avoid sausages, hot dogs, and meat covered in breadcrumbs*

Low-Carb Fruits

- Avocado should be your favorite fruit for the Keto Diet

- Other fruits detailed in the grocery list provided

Beverages and Condiments

- Lukewarm water, coffee, black or herbal tea

- Bone broth

- Fermented drinks like yogurt

- Lemon or lime juice

- Fruit juices (you can make a cocktail)

FOODS TO EAT MODERATELY

Vegetables and Mushrooms

- Nightshades such as eggplants and peppers

- Some cruciferous vegetables such as white and green cabbage, red cabbage, cauliflower, broccoli, Brussels sprouts, fennel, turnips

- Some root vegetables like spring onion, leek, onion, parsley root, garlic

- Mushrooms and winter squash (i.e., pumpkin)

- Sea vegetables such as nori and kombu

- Bean sprouts, sugar snap peas, wax beans, globe or French artichokes

- All varieties of berries—blackberries, blueberries, strawberries, raspberries, cranberries, mulberries

- Coconut, rhubarb, olives

Dairy Products

- Plain, full-fat yogurt

- Cottage cheese

- Heavy cream

- Sour cream

- Cheese

Nuts and Seeds

- Macadamia nuts

- Pecans, almonds, walnuts, hazelnuts

- Pine nuts, flaxseed, pumpkin seeds

- Sesame seeds, sunflower seeds, hemp seeds

- Brazil nuts (contain a very high level of selenium)

Fermented Soy Products

- Fermented soy products such as natto, tempeh, and tamari

- Green soybeans

- Unprocessed black soybeans

Condiments

- Healthy zero-carb sweeteners like stevia and Swerve

- Thickeners such as arrowroot powder and xanthan gum

- Puree, passata, ketchup

- Cocoa and carob powder, extra dark chocolate, cocoa powder

FOODS TO AVOID

Alcohol

- Dry red wine, dry white wine

- Spirits

- Beers

Instead, opt for low-carbs cocktail drinks

Foods with added sugars – They include artificial sugars and sweeteners that spike blood sugars. They are not suitable for ketosis and may have an adverse impact on your overall health.

Grains – A large variety of grains are rich in carbs which do not favor ketosis. Most grains have negligible or no amounts of fats. Grains such as wheat, rye, oats, corn, barley, millet, bulgur, sorghum, rice, amaranth, buckwheat, and sprouted grains should be avoided. Moreover, products made from grains should be avoided. They include pasta, bread, pizza, cookies, and crackers, among others.

Factory or farmed pork and fish – They contain highly inflammatory omega-6 fatty acids. Farmed fish contains mercury and polychlorinated biphenyl (PCBs). PCBs are organic chlorine compounds which increase the risk of various cancers like liver cancer and gallbladder cancer.

Processed foods – These foods contain a high amount of sugar additives and chemical preservatives which may alter ketosis. Furthermore, some include sulfites, which may negatively impact your overall health.

Milk – Only a very small amount of milk is recommended while on the Keto Diet. Of all dairy products, milk contains the highest amount of carbs. In fact, 100 ml of milk may have4-5 grams of carbs. Moreover, milk contains hormones (especially rBGH injected into dairy cows to boost milk production) which may destabilize digestion.

Sugary foods – It is prudent to note that each teaspoon of sugar has around ten grams of carbohydrates. This means that sugar intake is contrary to the Keto Diet, which dictates that carbohydrates should be consumed in small amounts.

Legumes – Most legumes are relatively high in carbs and should be avoided. Apart from peanuts, legumes such as beans, chickpeas, and lentils are rich in carbs. They are also linked to leaky gut syndrome, IBS, and Hashimoto's thyroiditis. Some people have shown no signs of these complications when they eat peanuts.

Note: The list of what you should eat might contain some foods with may irritate your stomach. Perhaps you are allergic to them. You should consult your dietician to get more advice concerning the foods you should avoid, even if they appear on the Keto Diet.

Complete Grocery List

The Keto Diet is effective only if dieters eat the right foods. You can't just go into a grocery store and buy anything. The Keto Diet's effectiveness is contingent on what dieters consume. That is why we track macros and stick to a certain menu plan. This section will help you know what you should buy to make keto meals.

The food list in this section is not only created to kick-start the Keto Diet. You can still eat most of these foods even when you enter ketosis. Any additional items in the ingredients listed here should be properly researched. There is a lot of misleading information about keto foods. Do not take such information seriously if you want your diet to be effective.

Below is a complete grocery list of keto food including vegetables, fruits, dairy products, meat, poultry, seafood, fats and oils, nuts and seeds, and spices and condiments.

Vegetables

When beginning the Keto Diet, it is imperative to note the vegetables that you should incorporate in your meals. Keto meal plans include vegetables, but in moderate amounts. This is because most vegetables contain a huge amount of carbs which are not favorable for ketosis.

Ideally, the best vegetables for the Keto Diet should contain more nutrients and low carbs. Such vegetables should be dark and leafy like kale and spinach. However, the vegetable list for the Keto Diet is not limited to just dark and leafy farm produce. Here is a list including most of the vegetables:

- Canned asparagus

- Avocado

- Bean sprouts

- Artichokes

- Canned black olives

- Asparagus

- Bok choy

- Broccoli

- Brussel sprouts

- Cabbage

- Bell peppers (green, red, yellow, orange)

- Canned artichoke Hearts

- Canned green beans

- Canned pickles

- Green onions

- Canned sauerkraut

- Eggplant

- Fresh spinach

- Canned green olives

- Romaine lettuce

- Canned greens

- Canned mushrooms

- Green bell peppers

- Portabella Mushrooms

- Radishes

- Greens

- Hot peppers

- Celery

- Cucumbers

- Iceberg lettuce

- Leeks

- Fresh mushrooms

- Canned spinach

- Cauliflower

- Napa cabbage

- Okra

- Spaghetti squash

- Snow peas

- Yellow onions

- Spinach

- Yellow squash

- Zucchini

Fruits

It is nutritious to include fruits in the Keto Diet. However, the intake of sugary fruits should be limited because they will increase glucose levels in the body. With that in mind, it is important to remember the ketosis process thrives on low glucose levels. Therefore, fruits should be consumed in small quantities. Fruits may limit the intake of artificial sweeteners since they quench your craving for sugar.

Fruits are also a good source of fiber, which helps the digestive system. Below is a list of fruits in line with Keto Diet standards:

- Blackberries

- Fresh cranberries

- Apricot

- Avocado

- Cherries

- Dates

- Apples

- Figs

- Grapes

- Kiwi

- Melons

- Nectarines

- Olives

- Lemons

- Limes

- Peaches

- Pears

- Grapefruit

- Guava

- Mango

- Oranges

- Papaya

- Raspberry

- Rhubarb

- Strawberries

- Passionfruit

- Tangerines

- Pineapples

- Plums

- Pomegranates

- All varieties of tomatoes

Dairy products

The Keto Diet is sensitive to dairy products. Many dairy products may have extremely high levels of fat which may be excess for ketosis. For this reason, dairy products should be consumed with proper knowledge of the fat content.

Dairy products cause some people to have stomach bloating, cramps, diarrhea, and nausea. In order to gradually get used to dairy products, you can add small quantities into your meals. However, it is wise to obtain alternative fat sources if you want to go keto and you happen to be sensitive to dairy products. Studies have shown that sensitivity to dairy products may be caused by a digestive system disorder called lactose intolerance. Certainly, dairy products contain lactose which causes an allergic effect.

Do not assume that any dairy product is keto friendly. Here is a list of the dairy products that you should consume while on the Keto Diet. Dairy products which do not appear on the list may be incorporated with caution in the Keto Diet.

Yogurts

- Mayonnaise

- Full fat/Full cream Greek yogurt

- Heavy whipping cream

- Sour cream

- Full fat/Full cream milk

Cheeses

- Cream cheese

- Monterey Jack

- Mozzarella

- Colby

- Blue

- String cheeses

- Swiss

- Brie

- Cheddar

- Cottage cheese

- Feta

- Goat cheese

- Parmesan

Meats

The Keto Diet includes low-carb-high-fat meats that are perfect for boosting ketosis. However, meat should be consumed with caution. Consuming large quantities of meat means more fat for ketosis. As it is, excess fats should be avoided at all times.

Additionally, more meat in the stomach means that more acids will be produced to aid digestion. In turn, high levels of acids may be corrosive to the stomach lining and can cause abdominal pains.

The following is a list of various types of meat that you can eat while on the Keto Diet. Ensure that you buy lean cuts of meat with a small amount of fat.

Organic processed meats (expensive) may also be adopted into keto meals. Meats are carb- free but organic processed meats may have some sugar from preservatives. Therefore, it is prudent to check the ingredients and make the right purchase decision.

Beef

- Prime rib

- Corned beef

- Roast beef

- Hamburger

- Steak

- Baby-back ribs

Organ meats (offal)

- Heart

- Liver

- Tongue

- Kidney

- Offal

Pork:

- Pork roast

- Pork chops

- Ground pork

- Ham (unglazed)

- Bacon

- Tenderloin

- Ham

Avoid consuming large quantities of the following meats:

- Bacon

- Sausages

- Hot dogs

- Jerky

- Italian sausage

- Lamb

- Pepperoni

- Lunch meats

Poultry

At times, you can alternate lean meats with poultry. Poultry meat comes from chicken, ducks, and turkey. Many people prefer poultry because it is delicious and softer than red meat.

Poultry is a good source of the fats necessary for ketosis. However, consuming poultry meat with wheat flour products, as many people do, will add more carbs on the meat. This is not favorable for ketosis. Eat plain poultry meat to maximize the level of fats. Moreover, do not remove the white fat layer which covers poultry meat; it's a good source of fats. You could rear some poultry as organically as possible and make a great keto meal for whenever you please. Below are various types of poultry meat for keto dieters.

Chicken

- Whole chicken

- Chicken breasts

- Cornish hens

- Chicken eggs

- Chicken thighs

- Chicken wings

- Chicken legs

- Chicken tenders

Turkey

- Whole turkey

- Ground turkey

- Turkey breast

- Turkey legs

Duck – Eggs and meat

Goose – Eggs and meat

Quail – Eggs and meat

Seafood

Different kinds of seafood are great sources of heart-healthy omega-3 fatty acids which are good for keto dieters. Although some seafood may cost you more than lean meat, it may be a good substitute. People who are allergic to lean red meat and poultry meat are advised to try seafood.

Even so, some seafood, like oysters and mussels, contain some carbohydrates and should be consumed with caution. Below is a variety of seafood that you should try when on the Keto Diet:

- Salmon and tuna

- Oysters (some carbs)

- Salmon

- Sardines

- Catfish

- Cod

- Shellfish

- Crabs

- Anchovies

- Bass

- Tilapia

- Trout

- Tuna fish

- Halibut

- Herring

- Lobster

- Scallops

- Flounder

- Haddock

- Shrimp

- Sole

Fats and Oils

There are natural fats and oils that may be consumed as part of keto meals. The majority of these fats and oils occur naturally in animals, fish, and plants. Even as they are helpful in enhancing ketosis, they should only be consumed in the specified amounts.

Many people are sensitive to fats and oils because they may not have a pleasant taste. You can start with small amounts and gradually increase as you get used to the taste. Generally, fats and oils are meant to be added to food in small, appropriate amounts. For example, you can sparingly add fat and oils to rice or use them as a topping for lean cuts of meat.

When buying vegetable oils such as olive, flax, or safflower oils, opt for cold-pressed oils if they are available. This is because they allow less oxidation, which means that you get more essential fatty acids. Additionally, you can use the fats and oils to fry your food.

Some Keto Diet foods that are good sources of fats and oils include:

- Tallow

- Avocados

- Non-hydrogenated animal fat

- Lard

- Coconut butter

- Egg yolks

- Macadamia/Brazil nuts

- Cocoa butter

- Mayonnaise

- Avocado oil

- Macadamia oil

- Coconut oil

- MCT Oil

- Béarnaise sauce

- Peanut oil

- Sesame oil

- Bacon fat

- Duck fat

- Ghee

- Hollandaise sauce

- Sunflower oil

Nuts and Seeds

Nuts and seeds are high-fat and low-carb foods which are heart-healthy, high in fiber, and may lead to healthier aging. They provide the body with up to eight grams of net carbs per ounce. Frequent consumption of nuts has been attributed to reduced risk of heart disease, certain cancers, depression, and other chronic diseases.

Additionally, they are great sources of fats that can enhance ketosis. They have fiber, which boosts digestive activities. What makes nuts and seeds perfect ingredients for the Keto Diet is that they have low net carbs and a high amount of fat.

Below are most of the nuts and seeds that one should incorporate in the Keto Diet:

- Almonds

- Brazil nuts

- Cashews

- Macadamia nuts

- Pecans

- Pistachios

- Walnuts

- Chia seeds

- Flaxseeds

- Pumpkin seeds

- Sesame seeds

Spices and condiments

People love spices and will go to any lengths to spice their food up. More than just making food delicious, spicing food improves your appetite. However, keto dieters should consume spices in moderation since most spices contain carbs. The more spices you add to your food, the more carbs you consume.

There are low-carb spices and condiments on the market that are highly recommended for keto dieters. Processed spices are not that favorable to ketosis. In fact, a handful of them include glycemic index sweeteners which should be avoided while on the Keto Diet. While seasoning food, keto dieters should quit using table salt and instead use sea salt which contains powdered dextrose.

When buying spices, ensure that you read the nutrition label to ensure they don't have added sugar. On the same note, did you know that black pepper contains carbs? It does! The number of carbs in spices is minimal, so consuming huge amounts of spices would be the only cause for alarm. Carbs may accumulate quickly and negatively impact ketosis.

Below are some of the common natural herbs and spices that you should use in Keto Diet meals:

- Rosemary

- Cilantro

- Parsley

- Cinnamon

- Cumin

- Mustard

- Horseradish

- Mayonnaise

- Oregano

- Thyme

- Ketchup

- Sauerkraut

- Salad dressings

- Relish

Food Quality

Food quality in the Keto Diet requires controlling the foods that you take in every meal, including the right amounts of macros. You must be vigilant to ensure that you track macros in every meal. Additionally, you must check the package label for processed keto meals to ensure that you are eating the right quality of foods.

Food quality in the Keto Diet is an easy thing. All you need to do is to eat the recommended foods and in the right amounts. It is important to avoid foods that are categorized as unhealthy in the Keto Diet. If anything, you should not even have any of those foods in your fridge. You will be tempted to eat a small amount and that will have an immense impact on ketosis.

Eating quality food during every keto meal will boost ketosis. Furthermore, you will be maintaining your health and enhancing your immune system. In short, food quality in the Keto Diet can be maintained by:

- Understanding the main foods to eat

- Eating the right amounts of macros

- Avoiding unhealthy foods

Make sure you follow standard sanitation practices for food preparation. Without proper sanitation, you may end up eating healthy foods which are contaminated.

Then the food's usefulness in the body will be negligible. In fact, consumption of healthy but dirty foods leads to food poisoning complications.

Manufacturers can also observe food quality by improving and sustaining basic quality standards. Reducing unhealthy components in processed foods is a great way to control food quality. Use of excess artificial ingredients in the processing of consumable foods is unethical. Such behaviors by manufacturers should be prosecuted and attract serious penalties.

Supplements That Go Well With the Keto Diet

While following the Keto Diet plan, you may incorporate some supplements. These supplements are meant to boost the levels of various macros in keto meals. This section highlights common supplements that may be consumed as part of the Keto Diet.

MCT Oils

Medium chain triglycerides (MCTs) are a type of fat molecule that naturally occurs in fat foods. Major sources of MTCs include coconut oil, palm oil, cheese, butter, and yogurt. It is possible for MCTs to be separated from other fatty acids and used as energy within a short while.

MCT shave a shorter chain length than other fatty acids and this makes them metabolize faster. When they are metabolized, they can effectively be converted to ketones and used for fuel. In short, MCTs are beneficial for boosting keto dieters' energy levels and facilitating continuous ketosis.

Vitamin D

Vitamin D is very important whether or not you are on the Keto Diet. The vitamin has a huge impact on your overall health. Many people have a deficit of Vitamin D and that is why it is advisable to take its supplements. They boost both immunity and electrolyte absorption. Moreover, Vitamin D assists in calcium absorption and enhances muscle functions. It naturally occurs in eggs yolks, fish oil, and mushrooms among other foods included in the Keto Diet. Nevertheless, the main natural source of Vitamin D is the sun. Basking in the sun during a warm morning would give you an immeasurable amount of Vitamin D.

Electrolytes

When transitioning from one diet to another, you may experience some body changes. One of the many changes is increased urination. Electrolytes such as sodium and potassium may be lost as part of the urine. Replenishing these electrolytes is important because they may solve some of the potential side effect of ketosis, like headaches and fatigue. Electrolyte supplements are easy to buy at pharmacies. However, caution should be taken when consuming electrolyte supplements. Taking more than the recommended amount may affect your metabolism.

Protein Powder

Protein powder is a high quality and convenient source of protein. However, many brands of protein powder contain sugar, which may not be favorable to ketosis. This means that even though protein powder is a great source of protein, it should be used sparingly. If you want to enter ketosis faster while consuming protein powder, choose one with low levels of sugar.

Omega-3 Fish Oil

There are many health benefits derived from eating fish. One of them is acquiring omega-3 oils which are essential in boosting health in any keto dieter. Fish oil in supplemental form provides a perfect ratio of omega-3 in its purest and most concentrated type. Basically, omega-3 improves the performance and growth of muscles in a healthy way. Additionally, omega-3 fatty acids support good blood circulation to allow nutrients to reach muscles.

Whey Protein

This protein supplement is without an equal. It has a high absorption rate in the body. Most pro trainers consume this supplement after exercising. It should also be incorporated in the Keto Diet as a key supplement. Ideally, keto dieters should take the supplement to round out the protein balance in the body.

Whey protein has a high biological value and is convenient to take at any time. Additionally, the whey protein supplement may be rapidly shuttled into the muscles as compared to protein obtained from food. This means that it can exert more powerful anabolic effects.

Branch-Chain Amino Acids (BCAA)

Keto beginners can improve the ketosis process if they start BCAA supplements. Muscles grow gradually and a noticeable improvement in muscle density is witnessed. BCAAs provide essential amino acids for muscle building. Chemically, they include leucine, isoleucine, and valine and they should be taken as components of the keto foods.

The three types of amino acids present in BCAAs are

important for recovery of muscle tissues. Additionally, they are essential in recovering proteins lost during hard training. As a primary muscle-building supplement, BCAAs should top every keto beginner's shopping list, especially if they want to lose weight.

Creatine

This supplement is well known among many pro trainers because it came into the market in the nineties. Athletes around the world use this supplement for a healthy and agile body. Recently, keto dieters have also developed an interest in the nutritional value of the supplement. Creatine supports the increase in energy in the body, as well as the size and strength of muscles. It has proven to have a long-term muscle-building effect.

Vitamins/Mineral Supplements

Multivitamins and mineral supplements support cellular conditions which in turn boost ketosis, performance, and muscle growth. The supplements contain compounds like Vitamins A, C, and E. These vitamins are called oxidants and are important for immune functions. Moreover, they cause synergistic effects which result in perfect health for keto dieters.

Risks of Taking Supplements

Just like other drugs, a dietary supplement may have risks and side effects on your body. Consider checking with your dietician to determine the right supplements for you. Many supplements are self-prescribed, with no prior informed medical advice from doctors, dieticians, or pharmacists.

Taking supplements at random and without information about the risks can be a fatal thing. It is worthwhile to note that there is a lot of information concerning supplements. To be safe, get advice from a certified and experienced expert in order to avoid the following risks associated with supplements.

Excess Supplement Settles in Your Arteries

Taking excessive supplements, with the aim of maximizing their benefits, may just cause complications. Excess supplements may accumulate inside your arteries. This may lead to clogging and lethal heart complications. High blood pressure and heart diseases are likely to occur.

Supplements Can Harm Your Kidneys

Multivitamin supplements provide the body with Vitamin D, which is healthy. However, there's a risk of absorbing too much Vitamin D into the kidneys. This is because an excess level of Vitamin D triggers extra calcium absorption, which leads to kidney stones.

Contamination

Taking dietary supplements carries the risk of possible contamination with harmful substances. Research has indicated that most supplements are contaminated with heavy metals such as mercury, cadmium, and lead. Additionally, over 40 percent of supplements may have pesticide residues. Toxicities from heavy metals are potentially life-threatening.

Drug Interactions

A lot of people are fond of taking over-the-counter drugs while taking supplements. This is risky since it can cause drug interactions. For example, taking supplements that contain Vitamin A while under Accutane medication (a prescription drug for the treatment of cystic acne) can increase the toxic effects of the drugs. Vitamins in the supplements can interfere with blood-thinning medications used to treat and prevent blood clots.

Keto Power Foods

Keto power foods are mainly meant for bodybuilders who require maximum energy. Some people think that a low-carb-high-fat diet will only make them obese. Without a doubt, that is a weird thinking. It is actually much easier to gain a different body shape while under the Keto Diet. Bodybuilding foods are mainly proteins and not fats. In actual sense, some people have to lose body fat to gain muscles.

However, the Keto Diet can enhance the loss of body fats and boost muscle building. Consuming fats in the Keto Diet plan is only meant to create a source of energy for the body and not to add more body fat. Therefore, you can opt for some keto power foods and still gain muscle. Keto power foods are meant to help you feel full as well as give you the power to endure your training sessions.

Here are examples of keto power foods.

- Steak and eggs – Both steak and eggs are rich in fats and proteins. Steak and two fried eggs can serve as perfect keto power foods. They provide the body fats for ketosis and protein for bodybuilding. The high levels of fats can be burned to produce maximum energy and body power.

- Chicken – Chicken meat is a great source of protein and fats. Like eggs and lean meat, chicken meat will boost your energy levels. This is the main reason chicken meat is included as a keto power food.

- Peanut butter shake – When you are looking for a keto power drink, you may want to add keto-friendly fruits and some peanut butter to make a shake. This will be a great source of energy, especially if eaten prior to a training session.

There are many keto power foods that can be prepared using the wide variety of ingredients listed as keto foods. You may consult your dietician to learn more about commonly recommend keto power foods.

Food Substitutes on the Keto Diet

The Keto Diet is very strict when it comes to meals. However, there is always room to make changes while sticking to healthy, low-carb-high-fat foods. It is important to know the substitutes for certain keto foods. Getting to know the available substitutes will enable you to develop a variety of recipes that can be used on the Keto Diet plan.

Here are some of the common substitutes for some Keto Diet foods.

Stevia for Sugar

Sugar is not favorable for the Keto Diet, due to the high levels of carbs it has. For any keto dieter, stevia is a good substitute for sugar. As mentioned earlier, stevia is a sweetener used as a sugar substitute and is extracted from the leaves of a plant in the stevia rebaudiana species.

Stevia gives you the same satisfaction as sugar. However, it is healthier because it does not contain calories. The major disadvantage with stevia is it may take a while to get used to the taste. Having some stevia twice a day is a great way to get used to it. Before you know it, you will be using stevia comfortably and without minding the taste.

Pork Rinds for Breadcrumbs

Sprinkling some breading on foods gives them an extra bit of goodness. The problem with breadcrumbs lies in the fact that they have high amounts of carbs. This makes it necessary to have substitutes to replace breadcrumbs. For this purpose, pork rinds are the best substitute. Pork rinds are low carb and, when crushed, they appear act exactly like breadcrumbs. You should not worry about an awful taste because pork rinds do not change the flavor of whatever you add them to.

Lettuces Leaves and Tortillas

Many people love tortillas. This makes it boring when they have to leave tortillas because they start the Keto Diet, but they do not have an option because tortillas contain a lot of carbs.

Lettuce is the best substitute for tortillas. Having some lettuce leaves in any meal will provide you with the same crunch as hard-shell tortillas. Lettuce has a negligible amount of carbs.

Almond Flour

Traditionally, white flour is a baking ingredient. It seems hard to find a substitute. Nonetheless, keto dieters can replace wheat flour with almond flour. Almond flour is made by grinding and processing almond seeds. Almond flour has significantly fewer carbs, high-fat levels, and more protein than normal flour. If you can't find almond flour, you can also use coconut flour.

Cauliflower Rice

Rice is one of those foods that some people like to have at every meal. The downside to rice is that it contains a lot of carbohydrates. If you want something similar to rice, you need to try cauliflower rice. They even look similar from a distance. The taste is pretty much the same. The only difference between cauliflower and rice may be the texture. Cauliflower rice is a good option that will be healthier for you when you are in ketosis.

Veggie Noodles for Pasta

Typically, pasta goes along with many of our daily meals. However, if you are going keto, you will have to abstain from pasta because it is rich in carbs. Since pasta is unfit for the Keto Diet, veggie noodles are the next best option.

The advantage of veggie noodles is that they are very simple to make. All you need is a vegetable spiralizer to create low-carb noodle-shaped pieces of vegetables.

Coconut Oils for Vegetable Oils

Many people think that vegetable oil is the best option for a carb-restricted diet. What they do not know is that there are other varieties of low-carb oils that can replace vegetable oils. Vegetable oils may cause a lot of problems, especially when heated and consumed. For this reason, the benefits of using coconut oils become more paramount.

Coconut Milk for Dairy Milk

Coconut milk is a perfect switch for dairy milk. It's low

carb and high-fat, which makes it suitable for the Keto Diet. There is not much difference between coconut milk and dairy milk. People who use powdered milk often can't tell the difference. Even though coconut milk may not be as creamy as whole milk, it serves the same purpose as milk.

Coconut oil has a lot of saturated fats, which are healthy and keto friendly. You will remain healthy for a long time while also cutting back on your intake of carbs. Moreover, saturated fats help the body in maintaining energy.

Cream Cheese Pancakes

Pancakes are a preferred breakfast by many people. In fact, many people would not complain if they had pancakes for every breakfast throughout the year. However, pancakes are not the best option for the Keto Diet. They are rich in carbs since they are made with wheat flour.

Cream cheese pancakes are a fantastic, healthy, keto-friendly stand-in. The taste will impress you and leave you wondering why you never knew about cream cheese pancakes before. Bulletproof Coffee for Coffee

It is obvious that many people like starting their day with a cup of coffee. However, coffee is not a great option for a Keto dieter. This is because of the sugar and cream you are likely to add to the coffee. Replacing the normal coffee with bulletproof tea is a great idea. It is simple to make and doesn't need sugar or cream. Due to this, many nutritionists advocate that Keto dieters should take bulletproof and avoid coffee at all cost.

Mashed Cauliflower for Mashed Potatoes

The best low carb substitute for mashed potatoes is mashed cauliflower. If made the right way, it is hard to tell the difference between mashed potatoes and mashed cauliflower. Making mashed potatoes is easier than mashed potatoes. Actually, most people like mashed cauliflower because there is no need to peel any potatoes. Moreover, the time taken to cook mashed cauliflower is much lesser than that taken to prepare mashed potatoes. In short, you get a super substitute for lesser time and effort.

Fathead Crust for Pizza Crust

Some people may not take it easy missing to taking pizza just because they are on the Keto diet. However, one can replace pizza crust with fathead crust to ensure that one does not sabotage the Keto diet. Fathead pizza is grain free and has low carb levels. Thus, it is safe and friendly to the Keto diet guidelines. The major drawback is that preparation of the fathead crust may take longer than pizza crust. It is worthwhile, especially if you are dying to have a piece of pizza. With fathead crust, one will realize that consuming pizza will not be regular.

The substitutes above are just a few examples to give you an idea. More information may be found online or from an expert in Keto Diet plans. Do not hesitate to research more keto-friendly substitutes to make your diet plan more interesting and easier to cope with.

Sweeteners in the Keto Diet

Most keto dieters develop sugar cravings. Sweeteners are the best sugar sources for the Keto Diet. It is okay to have some sugars even when you are on a Keto Diet. However, one should be cautious while using sweeteners because you may alter ketosis if you consume too much.

As a general rule, it is best to avoid sweeteners when starting the Keto Diet plan. When it comes to sugary items, anyone can be tempted to overeat. In turn, this can affect ketosis and the Keto Diet plan will have no impact. Therefore, stay strict about the use of sweeteners and try to consume only a few sweets when you develop a sugar craving.

The preferred sweeteners to use in the Keto Diet should have a low or insignificant amount Glycemic Index (GI). GI is the measure of how much a certain food raises the blood sugar. Many sweeteners have a GI of 0 (zero) which means that they do not raise blood sugar. Below are some types of 0-GI sweeteners that may sparingly be incorporated in the Keto Diet.

Stevia

Stevia is an herb that is also known as the sugar leaf. It has gained popularity among keto dieters and can be easily grown at home. Otherwise, you can purchase stevia in a grocery shop.

Allulose

This is one of the common low-calorie sweeteners on the market. It's made of monosaccharides, a simple sugar. Mostly, monosaccharide is found in wheat and fruits but in small quantities. Therefore, allulose may be made by processing wheat and some fruits. Despite allulose being a sugar, the body does not have the capacity to use it as fuel. This means that it is a healthy sweetener.

Inulin

Do not confuse insulin and inulin. Inulin is a natural sweetener that is extracted from chicory root. This type of sweetener may be absorbed by the body and should thus be consumed with maximum caution.

Monk fruit

This sweetener originated in China and is also known as Luo Han Guo. It is extremely sweet and one may have the tendency to eat more than required. In ancient China, traditional medicine men would use monk fruit to treat obesity and diabetes.

Erythritol

This sweetener is found in fruits and vegetables. It can be extracted from corn. Erythritol is a great sweetener because it does not affect blood sugar and has very few calories.

Alcohol in the Keto Diet

While on the Keto Diet, alcohol should be the least of your concerns. It is unfavorable to ketosis and should be avoided. This doesn't mean that you cannot enjoy a delicious drink or two on a special occasion. However, many alcoholic drinks contain a lot of sugar components. Consequently, this affects ketosis.

Reducing your consumption of beer and wine while on the Keto Diet is a great move. Consumption of alcohol has a number of effects on the liver and on metabolism.

As you drink, a high volume of ketones is produced. Frequently drinking a lot of alcohol is detrimental to liver metabolism. It may weaken the process of ketone creation. Below is a list of low-carb alcoholic drinks that and their impact on the to the Keto Diet.

Beer

Beer is a problem to the Keto Diet plan. There are immeasurable amounts of carbs in beer. Actually, some people call beer liquid bread because it's mostly made of wheat and sugar additives. For that reason, most beers are a disaster for the Keto Diet and should be avoided. If you must drink, research drinks which are keto friendly.

It is improper to mention any brands of beers that are keto friendly. Keto dieters need to look for information online and take time to scrutinize nutritional information in order to make well-informed choices.

Wines

You can incorporate a glass of wine even when you are on the Keto Diet. Wine is not a problem because a glass of wine contains less than 0.5 grams of sugar. Other sugar constituents in wine may be miscellaneous remains from the fermentation process. These sugar constituents do not have any effect on the blood sugar on insulin levels. All dry wines—dry white and red wines plus all unsweetened champagnes—fit into the Keto Diet.

Liquor

Despite being made from the fermentation of sugars, liquors do not have unhealthy carb level. Some dieticians suggest that liquors are the best choice of drink for keto dieters. They attribute this to the fact that most liquors are made from natural sugars. Drinking liquor in regulated amounts cannot negatively influence ketosis. However, you should avoid liquors if you are looking forward to losing weight on the Keto Diet. Liquors are known to hamper weight loss, especially if they contain high levels of sugar.

Spirits

When it comes to spirits, it is straightforward! They are the best alcohol drink to consume while on keto. Spirits like whiskey, brandy, and tequila have no carbs. However, spirits are the most dangerous drinks for the liver especially if consumed mindlessly. They may cause instant and irreversible damage.

Advice

The worst keto option is mixing alcohol with soda or

juice to make it less concentrated. This is equivalent to making a sugar bomb which will negatively impact ketosis.

There are plenty of people who report worse hangovers while on the Keto Diet. If you must drink, ensure you consume a lot of water to stay hydrated.

Lastly, *do not drink and drive*! It is inappropriate to put your life at risk.

Coconut Products for the Keto Diet

Coconut products are important constituents in keto meals. They contain high levels of healthy fats that are beneficial to the body even if someone is not the keto diet. Coconuts can make a variety of keto-friendly foods such as coconut milk, coconut cream, and coconut oil, among others. For instance, some dieticians suggest that coconut milk is a good alternative due to the presence of carbs in dairy milk. Most coconut products can be used as substitutes for most dairy products in equal amounts with a 1:1 ratio.

Below are the main coconut products recommended as being keto friendly.

Coconut Oil

Coconut oil is beneficial to the skin and oral health regimes. The best type of coconut oil is unprocessed and pure. When buying coconut oil, it is better to choose cold-pressed and centrifuge-extracted oil because it is creamy, smooth, and clear. Coconut oils can be added to sweet-savory keto baked foods, fried eggs, meats, and fish.

Coconut Butter

Coconut butter is similar to thick nut butter. It is made by grinding dehydrated coconut flakes using a food processor while adding small amounts of water. You can do it yourself at home. Coconut butter is rich in MCTs which are categorized as healthy keto fats. You can blend coconut oil into smoothies or spread them on slices of keto bread or low-carb pancakes.

Coconut Flour

Coconut flour is one of the best low-carb flours on the market. It makes tasty and low-carb baked foods that you can use as keto snacks. Foods made with coconut flour are satiating for a longer period than those made with wheat flour. Coconut flour is naturally low in digestible carbs and contains no gluten.

Coconut Vinegar

This coconut product provides a nice tang to recipes. It is fermented from the sap of a coconut tree. Typically, the fermentation process takes 45 to 60 days. It provides the keto dieter with beneficial bacteria which is naturally found in naturally fermented foods.

Coconut Cream

Coconut cream consists of healthy MCT oils which potentially boosts the immune system. You can also consume coconut cream in a cup of coffee.

Coconut Milk

Coconut milk is rich in flavor. It's made by pressing fresh coconut meat, is shelf stable, and can be stored for a long time compared to dairy milk.

Fermented Foods in the Keto Diet

Fermentation is a process in which bacteria or yeast is introduced to foods, juices, or milk products. As the process takes place, the microorganisms confuse the natural sugar elements present in the starting product. This leaves behind an acid or alcohol byproduct. The process has been used for thousands of years to preserve foods and drinks. Some common fermented foods are beer, wine, yogurt, and sourdough bread.

For the Keto Diet plan, it would be prudent to ignore alcohol and bread as they still remain rich in carbs. The healthy bacteria that should be consumed in fermented keto meals and drinks is known as lactobacillus acidophilus.

This is a "good" gut bacteria in the category of prokaryote bacteria. Lactobacillus acidophilus naturally occurs in the mouths and digestive tracts of human beings and most animals. This bacterium removes the natural sugars present in milk products, decaying fruits, and vegetables. Subsequently, it leaves behind lactic acid as the waste product. Lactic acid is useful in preserving foods and provides a typical sour taste to foods and drinks like yogurt.

Consuming fermented foods containing "good" bacteria, whether or not we are on keto, helps the digestive system to break down certain types of foods. It also goes a long way to prevent the growth and colonization of other bacteria that may be harmful to the digestive system.

Fermented keto foods should be unpasteurized. Pasteurization kills the bacteria, which renders the foods useless and unhealthy. Fermentation is preservative in nature and lowers the risks of bacterial infection from consuming unpasteurized fermented foods. If one wishes to ferment any foods for the Keto Diet plan, it is important to follow acceptable fermenting guidelines. This will ensure that no step is omitted and will reduce the chances of growing harmful organisms in the food.

Examples of fermented foods for the Keto Diet are yogurt, milk kefir, hard cheeses, fruit chutneys, and fermented vegetables. Some vegetables that can be fermented include beets, carrots, sauerkraut, pickles, and cabbages. Fermented cabbage juice is suggested to reduce intestinal gas, which causes stomach bloating.

Salt in the Keto Diet

When ketosis begins, you are likely to urinate more than usual over the first few weeks. As a result, you may lose most of the water retained in the body. Dissolved salts and minerals are flushed out along with the lost water. For the first few weeks, replacing the lost water, salts, and minerals is a crucial thing. Dehydration complications can arise if these important elements are not replenished. In fact, dehydration is the major cause of the keto flu and any other miserable feeling during the first weeks of switching to the Keto Diet.

It is healthy to continually consume water and salts for the period you remain on the Keto Diet. Dieticians suggest consuming as much as 3500-5000mg of salt in a day. However, keto dieters should not eat raw salt but salt which has cooked or boiled in food. Dietary changes, including water and salt intake while on the Keto Diet, should be discussed at length with a nutritionist. This is because a slight change in the intake of water and salts may cause adverse impacts on the effectiveness of the Keto Diet.

Salt is important, as it facilitates the liver's breaking down of fat into ketones. Also, salt (NaCl) is used in the production of stomach acid (HCl). So, how is salt associated with curbing the diseases that the Keto Diet may inhibit, such as blood pressure?

According to a recent study, lower salt intake was found to have a dramatic improvement on blood pressure. Another study carried out in the Dietary Approaches to Stop Hypertension (DASH), different levels of salt intake have an impact on the control of blood pressure. For instance, low salt intake reduces blood pressure while high salt intake spikes high blood pressure.

However, lowering salt intake may have a dire impact on worsening the total cholesterol to density lipoprotein (HDL) ratio. Therefore, low-density lipoprotein (LDL) becomes rampant and can lead to the heart disease. Triglycerides and insulin are also increased by lowering salt intake. Even as blood pressure stabilizes, your overall health may deteriorate when you lower salt intake below certain recommended levels.

So, what is the best level of salt to consume while on keto? The best answer to that may be answered in a diagnosis to determine your blood pressure. Your blood pressure levels may indicate how much salt you should consume.

Keto flu and salt intake

Keto flu is a major indication of sodium deficiency. The decrease in carb intake while on the Keto Diet leads to a drastic reduction in insulin levels. In turn, glucagon levels go up and the liver starts producing negatively-charged ketone bodies.

The negatively-charged ketone bodies pull positively-charged sodium ions out in the urine. This leads to salt depletion and causes the symptoms known as keto flu.

While on the Keto diet, one should be cautious in choosing the right type of salt. Commonly, the most recommended salts are natural salts. They are unprocessed and contain negligible amounts of impurities. It is advisable to get more information from your dietician about the right salt choices.

Good Fats vs. Bad Fats on the Keto Diet

Fats should be more than 70 percent of ingredients of a keto meal. Even as the Keto Diet advocates for the intake of more fats, not all fats are suitable for ketosis. It is important to know the type of fats you are consuming in order to avoid end up hurting your health with unhealthy fats.

This section provides a detailed comparison between good fats and bad fats on the Keto Diet.

Good Fats

Good fats which should be incorporated in the Keto Diet are saturated fats, monounsaturated fats (MUFAs), polyunsaturated fats (PUFAs), and naturally-occurring trans fats. These fats are healthy and will boost ketosis.

Saturated Fats

In the past, we were told not to consume saturated fats because they cause high- cholesterol-related health complications such as heart disease. However, recent research has debunked this notion and indicated that there is no link between saturated fats and heart disease.

Medium-chain triglycerides (MCTs) are examples of saturated fats which are healthy to consume. They are easily digested and used in ketosis. MCTs naturally occur in coconuts and in small amounts in butter and palm oil. They have numerous health benefits:

- Improved fat loss and athletic performance

- Improved HDL cholesterol levels and HDL to LDL ratio

- Enhanced and maintained bone density

- Boosted overall immune system

- Improved creation of important hormones like cortisol and testosterone

Here are the recommended types of saturated fats while on the Keto Diet:

- Red meat

- Cocoa butter

- Eggs

- Palm oil

- Lard

- Butter

- Cream

- Coconut oil

Monounsaturated Fats

Monounsaturated fatty acids (MUFAs) have been embraced by many diet plans as healthy for many years. Nutritionists link this type of fat to good cholesterol, which enhances ketosis.

Below are the health benefits of monounsaturated fats:

- Better insulin resistance.

- Increased HDL cholesterol levels

- Lowered blood pressure

- Lowered risk for heart disease

- Reduced belly fat

The following are common types of monounsaturated

fats for the Keto Diet:

- Olive oil

- Goose fat

- Lard and bacon fat

- Avocado and avocado oil

- Macadamia nut oil

Polyunsaturated Fats

Polyunsaturated fats are considered healthy fats. However, one should be cautious and avoid high volumes of this type of fats. Studies conducted on polyunsaturated fats indicated that they can form free radicals when heated. Free radicals are harmful compounds that increase inflammation along with carrying a risk of cancers and heart disease. Therefore, polyunsaturated fats are only safe and healthy if consumed when cold and should not be used for cooking. Polyunsaturated fats are very rich sources of omega-3 and omega-6 nutrients which are important to the body.

Health benefits of polyunsaturated fats include:

- They contain both omega-3 and omega-6, which have been associated with reduced risk of heart disease, stroke, and inflammatory diseases.

- They help improve symptoms of depression

Major sources of polyunsaturated fats are:

- Avocado oil

- Walnuts

- Fatty fish and fish oil

- Extra virgin olive oil

- Chia seeds

- Nut oils

- Flaxseeds and flaxseed oil

- Sesame oil

Natural Trans Fats

The only type of trans fats that should be included in keto meals is vaccenic acid. They naturally occur in grass-fed animal meats and dairy products. Most trans fats are harmful and unhealthy. Therefore, be cautious.

Here are the common health benefits of vaccenic acid:

- Reduced risk of heart disease, diabetes, and

obesity

- Possible reduction of cancer risk

The following are major sources of recommended types of natural trans fats:

- Grass-fed animal meats

- Dairy fats like butter and yogurt

Bad Fats

Most bad fats are processed and not in natural form. They contain unhealthy components which may cause life-threatening health complications. It is imperative to understand the main types of bad fats and avoid them at all times. The common types of bad fats are processed trans fats and polyunsaturated fats.

Processed Trans Fats and Polyunsaturated Fats

Processed trans fats are the types of bad fats that most people are aware of. They can be very damaging to your health and will disrupt your Keto Diet plans. Artificial fats that may be formed during food production are processed polyunsaturated fats.

Risks of consuming processed trans and polyunsaturated fats include:

- Reduced HDL (good) cholesterol and increased LDL (bad) cholesterol

- Increased risk of heart-related diseases

- Increased risks of cancer

- Inflammatory complications

Examples of trans fats to avoid include:

- Hydrogenated oils found in processed products such as cookies, crackers, margarine, and fast foods

- Processed vegetable oils like sunflower, safflower, cottonseed, soybean, and canola oils

Using Keto Fats and Oils

The Keto Diet is predominantly made up of fats. For this reason, keto dieters should know how to use each type of fats and oil to make the Keto Diet effective. You may take a walk through the grocery store and see vegetable oils, nut oils, seed oils, and olive oils. However, not all fats are created equal. Some go through intense processing before they are released to the market. Others are naturally extracted and are much healthier than processed ones. So what are the best oils and fats, and how should they be used? In other words, what are the nutritional functions of the main oils and fats used in the Keto Diet?

Below is a guide to various Keto Diet fats and oils:

Coconut Oil

Coconut oil is made up of MCTs which are known to boost metabolism and stimulate ketosis. The oils contain concentrated lauric acid that creates a longer shelf life. Coconut oil is also known to have antibacterial and antifungal benefits to the body. Like extra virgin olive oil, coconut may only be used in low-heat cooking.

Due to the high composition of saturated oils, coconut oils can be termed unhealthy. However, in recent years, studies have found that saturated fats reduce the risk of heart disease. For this reason, coconut oil has gained popularity among keto dieters and other people who are not necessarily on the diet. It has emerged as a super oil.

Olive Oil

Olive oil tends to be more popular than other oils because it has multiple health benefits, attributed to polyphenolic compounds. These compounds have antioxidants and anti-inflammatory effects on the body and reduce the risk of developing atherosclerotic plaques. In addition, studies have indicated that oleic acid, a component of olive oil, leads to a reduction of inflammatory contributors in the body.

Olive oils should not be cooked. Subjecting olive oil to high temperature causes it to lose its antioxidant and anti-inflammatory compounds.

Typically, extra virgin olive oil is primarily composed of monounsaturated fatty acids. It is processed and packed with antioxidants and has a robust flavor. Because of its low smoke point, extra virgin olive oil can be used in recipes that require a low simmer, like vegetables. Alternatively, the oil may be used as a salad dressing in keto meals.

Butter

If consumed in the right amounts, butter goes a long way in increasing vitamins A, D, and E in the body. Additionally, it boosts sodium butyrate and conjugated linoleic acid (CLA), which has anti-cancer properties. Most dieticians suggest that organic, free-range, grass-fed butter is generally more nutritious and does not contain antibiotics.

Regular butter has a low smoke point and should not be used in cooking. Instead, butter can be used with keto foods in its natural form. Otherwise, organic, grass-fed ghee may be used for high-heat cooking.

Grapeseed Oil

Grapeseed oil is rich in polyunsaturated fatty acids and may be obtained as a byproduct of winemaking. The main advantage of grapeseed oil is that it has a high smoke point and can be used in high-heat cooking. It has a great taste which makes it suitable for preparing foods without drowning out their flavor. Many restaurants use grapeseed oil because it is cheaper than olive oil.

However, grapes seed is not one of the healthiest cooking oils for keto meals because it is rich in omega-6 fatty acids. This reduces the omega-3 to omega-6 ratio in the body and may increase the risk of inflammation. In short, it is not healthy to consume more omega-6 than omega-3. Many people do not find it prudent to use grapeseed oil.

Peanut Oils

Peanut oil has vitamin E, which is an antioxidant which has a huge positive impact on controlling the risk of heart disease and cancer. Peanut oil may be used for deep frying because of its high smoke point. It remains the best option for keto dieters because it contains more than 30 percent healthy polyunsaturated fatty acids. The only downside is that it contains high levels of omega-6 fatty acids.

Avocado Oils

In a close comparison, avocado oil is similar to olive oil. It has a high level of monounsaturated fats, which are deemed to be healthy. Moreover, avocado oil contains a healthy dose of antioxidants whose health benefits are now known to us. Unlike olive oil, avocado oil has an extremely high smoke point. Therefore, the oil may be used in high-heat cooking. Avocado oil may be used for sautéing, frying, roasting or searing. The most common reason why keto dieters prefer avocado oil is because it is in liquid form at room temperature. Thus, it can be used in salad dressings and vinaigrettes.

Ghee

Ghee is one of the most preferred types of fats for the Keto Diet. It may be used for high-heat cooking because of its high smoke level. This means that ghee may be used in the preparation of high-temperature keto meals such as sautéing, frying, and baking. Separations of milk solids from butter give ghee a longer shelf life. Normally, ghee does not need refrigeration.

It is imperative for you to do your research and determine what fats and oils are best for you. Remember, your body may react differently as compared to another person. This means that a specific oil or fat may be good for one person and can cause havoc in the stomach of another. Just take care while using fats and oils at all times.

Whole-Food Fats

Whole food fats (WFF) are healthy fats and are considered keto friendly. They provide keto dieters with healthy fats that enhance ketosis. According to dieticians, whole food fats should be consumed freely and without a doubt of whether or not they are healthy. Whole foods fats are not anything new since they are mentioned in another section of the book.

Basically, whole food fats include monounsaturated fats, polyunsaturated fats, and saturated fats.

Monounsaturated Fats

This category of whole-food fats reduces the risk of heart disease and lowers cholesterol levels. The major fats include olive oil, avocado oils, and nut and seeds oils.

Polyunsaturated Fats

The two commonly known types of polyunsaturated fats are omega-3 and omega-6 fatty acids. Omega-3 fatty acids are known to provide anti-inflammatory effects. Additionally, they help to protect against heart disease and improve brain function. The main sources of polyunsaturated fats are cold-water fish such as salmon, tuna and trout, butter, eggs, coconut oil, nuts and seeds, chicken meat, and lean meat from grass-fed animals.

Saturated Fats

Saturated fats increase HDL-cholesterol levels in the body. In turn, HDL cholesterol reduces the bad cholesterol and fatty acids by transporting them to the liver for further processing. If not broken down into body-friendly fats, the unhealthy fats are excreted. The major sources of saturated fats are red meat, butter, coconut oil, and cheese.

How to Go Dairy-Free on Keto

You can avoid dairy products and still be successful on the Keto Diet. After all, most dairy products contain high carbs and more proteins than fats. Many people have dairy intolerances, whether or not they are on the Keto Diet. Below is a list of the dairy products that you should do away with while on keto:

- Cottage cheese

- Curds

- Butter and byproducts such as butterfat, butter oil, butter acid, butter esters, and buttermilk

- Casein, casein hydrolysate, rennet casein, and caseinates

- Lactalbumin, lactalbumin phosphate, and lactoferrin

- Cheese

- Heavy cream

- Milk-based protein powders

- Sour cream, sour cream solids, and sour milk solids

- Custard and pudding

- Lactose, lactulose, and tagatose

- Milk (in all forms animal milk)

- Whey (in all forms)

- Artificial butter flavor

- Caramel candies

- Chocolate

- Margarine

Instead, substitute the dairy products above with keto-friendly foods that provide the same satiety and satisfaction:

- Plant-based oils like coconut oil, tallow, and duck fat.

- Red meat, poultry, and seafood

- Leafy/green low-carb vegetables

- Low-carb fruits such as avocados, berries, and some citrus fruits

- Nuts and seeds

Here is a strategy on how to go dairy-free on keto:

- Reduce your dairy consumption to a point where you do not affect ketosis.

- Limit the specific forms of dairy that you are allergic to. Otherwise, take lactase enzyme together with your dairy-rich meal to reduce lactose intolerance.

- Eliminate small quantities of dairy products from your keto meals.

How to Go Grain-Free on Keto

Most grains are not keto friendly due to their high levels of carbs. Additionally, grains contain more proteins than fats. Therefore, you must eliminate grains from breakfast, snacks, lunch, and dinner.

Grains that should be avoided include wheat (and wheat products like bread), quinoa, barley, oats, corn, millet, rice, rye, amaranth, sprouted grains, and buckwheat. They are known to contain over 95 percent carbs and proteins, with negligible fats.

It is possible for keto dieters to go without grains. Any cravings for grains may be satisfied by eating nuts and seeds. The best nuts and seeds to consume include macadamia nuts, Brazil nuts, pecans, walnuts, almonds, peanuts, hazelnuts, pine nuts, pistachios, and cashew nuts. Additionally, any other types of nuts and seeds categorized as sources of healthy fats may be used as a grain substitute.

Chapter Four

Potential Side Effects of

Ketosis

This section will elaborate upon the side effects of ketosis and will offer some remedies. The side effects are "potential" since only 1 in 10 people on the Keto Diet may experience the side effects. Dieticians argue that the potential side effects are not lethal but do cause some discomfort.

When you suddenly switch your body metabolism from burning carbs to fats and ketones, you may have some side effects as the body adapts accordingly. Symptoms may include headaches, tiredness, muscle fatigue, cramping, and heart palpitations. The side effects are mild and short-lived for most people—at most for the first three weeks.

Every side effect has a unique solution. However, one of the major ways to gradually cut back on the side effects is to gradually reduce the consumption of carbs over the first few weeks of ketosis. This helps the body as its systems try adapting to fats as their primary source of energy as opposed to glucose.

Below are the most common possible side effects people may feel while entering ketosis.

Keto flu

The keto flu is common among beginners of the Keto Diet and typically occurs within the first week. It goes away after a short while of continuously being on the diet. Keto flu is mostly characterized by fatigue, headache, light nausea, inability to focus (brain fog), lack of motivation, and dizziness. There are a few reasons why the keto flu manifests itself in beginner keto dieters.

First, keto is diuretic. This means that the fluids retained in the body are lost as the body starts burning fats. Frequent urination leads to the loss of electrolytes. Water and electrolytes lost are vital to body functions and losing them makes you feel sick.

Secondly, the body is transitioning. Generally, the body is equipped to process a high intake of carbs as a source of energy. However, the keto diet reduces carbs and maximizes the intake of fats to commence ketosis. In turn, this forces the body to abruptly create enzymes to aid the transition. During this transition period, you are likely to experience things like nausea and headaches.

Solution

- The keto flu occurs as a result of dehydration and loss of salts. You can eliminate the flu by drinking sufficient water and salts. Also, drink two to three cups of bone broth (soup made from boiling fresh bones) twice per day.

Constipation

The number one reason for constipation is dehydration. As indicated above, ketosis may lead to a rapid fluid loss. Constipation can be very painful and may cause bruises around the anus. Without proper remedies, continued bruises may even lead to a wound around the anus.

Solution

- A simple solution to the constipation problem is increasing your water intake. You can drink between eight and 12 glasses per day. To kill two birds with one stone, you can put some salt in the water.

- Eat plenty of vegetables and other sources of fiber. Getting enough fiber in a diet keeps the intestines moist and this reduces the chances of constipation. It is worth it to note that a keto diet avoids fiber intake. Therefore, eating plenty of non-starchy vegetables may be a valid solution.

- You can use psyllium husk powder as a fiber supplement by dissolving it in drinking water.

Some people recommend milk of magnesia as another option to relieve constipation.

Low Alcohol Tolerance

When in ketosis, you tend to get intoxicated faster than usual because your body cannot tolerate alcohol as usual. This makes it necessary to lower your alcohol intake by at least half.

The reason for this common experience is still unclear. However, most dieticians believe that it is because the liver is busy burning fats to produce ketones and glucose. Due to this, the liver has less capacity to spare for processing alcohol.

On the other hand, this low alcohol tolerance could be because alcohol and sugar are broken down in almost the same way in the liver. Since the Keto Diet reduces sugar intake, the liver may become temporarily less adapted to processing sugars. Thus, the liver is also less adapted to processing alcohol. **Solution**

- Do not drink alcohol at all if you have not ascertained the macros present. Don't just drink any type of alcohol while on the Keto Diet. Take time to understand whether or not the alcohol in question is Keto friendly. If not just leave it and get going. Isn't ketosis a great moment to save your money?

Elevated cholesterol

Many studies indicate that cholesterol levels may increase during the Keto Diet. However, the most predominant type of cholesterol that is produced is HDL cholesterol which is also known as "good cholesterol." Good cholesterol lowers the chance of developing heart-related diseases.

People who want to lose weight may witness an increase in triglyceride counts. This enhances weight loss. Only a small percent of keto dieters may experience increased LDL cholesterol levels.

Solution

- Only eat when hungry – This may be helpful in reducing the quantity of fats consumed. Also, intermittent fasting will prove successful in curing elevated cholesterol levels.

- Consider using unsaturated fats like olive oil, fatty fish, and avocados. These types of fats are not harmful and will lower cholesterol levels in the body.

- Seek advice from your dietician or nutritionist about whether you should follow a strict low-carb-high-fat diet for health reasons. You will be less likely to have high cholesterol levels.

Hair loss

Hair loss is a rare experience and uncommon to the Keto Diet. However, we cannot rule out the possibility of its occurrence fora few Keto dieters. If it happens, there is no need to panic. It is a temporary condition with negligible hair loss. Ideally, it doesn't leave you with a bald head.

Solution

- Do not restrict calorie intake.

- Reduce as much stress as possible during your first few weeks on the Keto Diet.

- Get enough sleep.

- Do not simultaneously start an intense training program and the Keto Diet.

Keto rash

Some people start to itch when they start the Keto Diet. The keto rash is an irritation caused by acetone that is excreted through sweating. It is mainly experienced during the first few days of the Keto Diet

Solution

- Consider wearing clothing that absorbs sweat. Avoid nylon clothes at all times.

- Shower right after an activity that causes you to sweat.

- . If the problem persists, increase the carbs in your meals as well and change your exercise plans.

Cramps

Cramps, especially leg cramps, are common in beginners of the Keto Diet. They usually occur in the morning or at night. They're a major indicator of a mineral deficiently. Primarily, a lack of magnesium minerals causes cramps. Evidently, being in a low carb diet affects the levels of insulin which stimulates the kidneys to retain sodium minerals. Therefore, kidneys can no longer retain enough sodium levels which can lead to leg cramps. Also, when you are not consuming fruits rich in potassium and other nutrients, leg cramps may become rampant.

Solution

- Drink a lot of fluids and ensure you get enough

salt. This solves the magnesium deficit and prevents leg cramps.

- Try magnesium supplements. Ask your doctor about healthy and Keto friendly supplements that will help to mitigate cramps.

Heart palpitations

Most beginner keto dieters report an increase in their heartbeat. This is a common side effect during the transition period. It is not heart disease; your heart is just beating faster and harder and you should not get worried.

Solutions

- The preferable solution is to drink a lot of fluids and enough salt. This is an ideal and quick way to eliminate the problem.

- Try to avoid stress because it is a major result of the release of stress hormones, which make the problem worse.

- Slightly increase carb intake during your keto meals.

- If the problem persists, take potassium supplements once per day.

Reduced physical performance

A reduction in energy during the first few days of adapting to the Keto Diet may cause a decrease in physical performance. As the body shifts from using glucose to fat as a source of energy, all your strength and endurance may lessen. However, endurance and strength levels return to normal within a few weeks, after the body has fully adapted to the Keto Diet.

Solution

- Boost your intake of carbs before working out.

- Drinking a lot of water 30 minutes before exercising can make a huge difference.

Gallstones

Studies have been carried out to determine the link between the Keto Diet and gallstones. The findings are that gallstones may be among the side effects of the Keto Diet due to the lack of carbs.

Solution

- The best way to deal with this problem is to gradually increase fat intake to allow the body to adap faster.

Indigestion

Generally, switching to the Keto Diet eliminates indigestion and heartburn. However, indigestion is worse in the first week of starting the Keto Det. This is caused by the process of the body trying to adapt to a new diet. It is not a big problem and ends within the first week.

Solution

- Try to reduce fat intake in the first few days of the Keto Diet. Afterward, gradually increase the amount of fats as your body gets used to the diet.

Dragon breath

Most people who cut their carb intake to remain in ketosis may develop distinctive and bad breath nicknamed "dragon breath." The odor starts out sweet, similar to a fruity smell. Typically, the smell originates from acetone, a ketone compound. It is a sign that the body is burning lots of fat and converting ketones to body fuel. However, the smell turns nasty especially when working out and sweating a lot.

It is important to note that not everyone who starts the

Keto Diet experiences dragon breath. Even in those who do, it is temporary and goes away within a week or two. After two to three weeks, the body is fully adapted to the Keto Diet and ketones stop leaking through breathing or sweating.

Solution

- Drink a lot of fluids. As you enter ketosis, you become dehydrated. This means you need to drink more water and increase the volume of saliva to wash away the bacteria developing inside your mouth.

- Maintain good oral hygiene by brushing your teeth regularly. Otherwise, you can use breath refreshers.

- Reduce the degree of ketosis by reducing the amounts of fats you eat. Additionally, eating a higher amount of carbs can reduce the ketosis rate. Intermittent fasting is also another viable solution to regulate ketosis.

- If nothing seems to work, just be patient and give your body time to get used to the metabolism changes. Anyway, the bad breath is for a short period.

Insomnia

Insomnia is a difficulty sleeping, staying asleep, or a pattern of chronic poor sleep. Mainly, doctors attribute the problem to mental states such as anxiety, stress, and depression. Other factors that contribute to insomnia are hormonal imbalances and change of lifestyles like eating habits, illnesses, and medical disorders.

The relationship between insomnia and ketosis is not fully understood. However, some dieticians think that is all about the change in dietary patterns. Insomnia may be a long-term problem if not dealt with. This may cause extreme weight loss, even to an undesired level. It is prudent to get the help of a medical expert concerning insomnia the first time you experience it.

Solution

- Get a massage. Additionally, you may visit an acupuncture expert and get some magic from the needles.

- If the problem persists, see your personal doctor for a diagnosis of any underlying issues.

Acne

Keto dieters may, from time to time, experience acne,

especially on the face. Many people suggest that acne on the face is caused by an abnormal accumulation of fatty compounds underneath the skin. Mostly, this happens as the fatty elements are being excreted through the skin. However, they do not occur in everyone doing the Keto Diet.

Solution

- Stay hydrated – This helps to dissolve the fatty compounds and eliminates the unwanted levels as part of sweat.

Exfoliate – Cleaning the pores of your skin enhances healthier sweating.

Increased Sugar Cravings

Some people experience carbohydrate cravings it the first few weeks into the Keto diet plan. This is due to a blood sugar response from lack of sufficient carbs intake. Others may exhibit a strong craving for sugar during the transition period. However, it is good to stick to the Keto diet guidelines and abstain from taking sugary foods. After all, the craving is short-lived – usually common within the first 2 days to the second week of the Keto diet plan. The good news is that some beginners do not experience cravings.

Solution

Even as one may be on the strict Keto diet, it may be inevitable to satisfy the craving with little amounts of sugar. However, this should strictly be the healthy sugar substitutes listed in this book.

Risks of Kidney damage

During ketosis, the body loses a lot of electrolytes and fluid due to urination. The loss of electrolytes such as sodium, potassium, and magnesium can increase the risk of acute kidney problems. According to various doctors, dehydration is a serious disorder which may result in kidney stones and severe kidney injuries. Additionally, this may put a Keto dieter at risk of cardiac arrhythmia as electrolytes are necessary for a normal beating of the heart. Irregular heartbeats may lead to heart complications.

Solution

- One should take enough water volumes to stay hydrated during the Keto diet. Dehydration can only be tackled by consuming enough water, usually deemed to be not less than 8 glasses per day.

- Dieticians may be consulted about the best supplements for the electrolytes lost.

Dizziness and Drowsiness

Due to the loss of water and electrolytes, a Keto dieter may feel dizzy and lightheadedness. However, these are not fatal symptoms as they are avoidable.

Solutions

- Eat foods that are rich in potassium such as leafy greens, broccoli, and avocados among others

- Add enough salt to foods or use salty broth when cooking

- Take supplements with a directive from an expert. For example, magnesium citrate is an example of a good magnesium supplement.

Low Blood Sugar

Low blood sugar is a common side effect in many keto diet beginners. It is also termed as hypoglycemia. It often occurs when glucose in the body is lower than the required levels. This can make a dieter feel a temporary hunger and fatigue.

Solution

- Tracking macros to ensure enough carbs are in the diet can go a long way in solving low blood sugar.

- On the other hand, there are sugar substitutes that may provide the body with sufficient glucose while still sticking to Keto diet guidelines.

Diarrhea

On the flip side of the previously mentioned side effect of constipation, some people may experience minor diarrhea issues in the first few days of Keto diet. This is simply due to the body adjusting to the macro ratio changes. For instance, limiting the intake of carbs and increasing proteins and fats can lead to diarrhea.

Solution

- Ensure that carbs are sufficiently replaced by full-fat source instead of proteins.

Take a teaspoon of psyllium husk powder or sugar-free Metamucil before eating any meal. This will really improve the situation.

Why the Keto Diet Is Not Working For You

Many beginners start the Keto Diet with eagerness to achieve the desired health benefit. However, time might pass and nothing seems to happen, including weight loss. Obviously, you are adapting to the Keto Diet, but if you are not witnessing any changes, this can be very frustrating. There are various reasons that may be responsible for this drawback.

You are not in ketosis

You might assume that you're in ketosis even as there are no signs related to the start of the process. There is a need to measure your ketone levels. You can test for ketosis using the various methods listed in a prior section this book. Just as a quick reminder, the methods are:

- Urine strips

- Breath testing

- Blood testing (the most accurate)

Once you find out that you are not in ketosis, visit your dietician for advice. The bottom-line may be to increase fat intake to boost ketosis.

You are not monitoring hidden carbs

The Keto Diets aims to minimize your intake of carbs. If you are not cautious and often include high amounts of vegetables, dairy products, and nuts in your meals, you are spoiling the Keto Diet. These are items that most people consume, unaware that they contain high amounts of carbs.

Nuts are known to be a satiating food which may be eaten as part of a snack. However, people make the mistake of consuming more than required. They increase carbs in the diet and thus impact the Keto Diet.

Other hidden carbs are found in vegetables including cabbage, cauliflower, broccoli, fennel, and turnips. You should limit the intake of these vegetables at all times to make the Keto Diet more effective. Additionally, limit your consumption of fruits since they contain high amounts of sugars.

You have leptin resistance

Leptin is a fat-controlling hormone that notifies the brain when you are satiated. In other words, leptin tells the brain when the stomach is full and you need to stop eating. It regulates the amount of fat we carry in the body.

Leptin resistance means that you have enough hunger

hormones but the messages about being satiated are not being transferred to the brain. This is a disaster which can easily lead to fatal overeating.

Obese people actually have enough leptin. The problem is that leptin sends messages but they aren't registered properly by the brain. Thus, one continues to eat even when he should actually stop.

You are eating too much fat

Despite the fact that the Keto Diet requires fats to be the dominant dietary ingredient, you must know the acceptable levels. Eating extremely high levels of fat thinking that you are supporting ketosis is a mistake. Do not forget that fats contain twice the level of calories as proteins. Eating more fats than necessary may cause excessive caloric consumption which curtails ketosis. Regardless of how fast you may want results from the Keto Diet, it is advisable to stick to the maximum levels of fats as dictated by your dietician. Note that if you are not eating the right amounts of fats, the Keto Diet will only frustrate your health-related goals.

You have food sensitivities

Have you done all that is required in adhering to macros and tracking but still do not feel any change? You may have food sensitivity issues. Food sensitivity is a propensity to be affected by a particular category of foods. Many people call the disorder an allergy. For example, one may be sensitive to meat, meaning that he is more likely to be sensitive to proteins. A large group of people may have this problem with dairy products such as cheese, cream, yogurt, ghee, and butter.

When you are food sensitive, you are not able to eat some of the foods suggested by the Keto Diet plan. Instead, you end up looking for substitutes which may not contain the same macro levels compared to the suggested foods. Definitely, this will affect how effective the Keto Diet is for you.

You are not eating sufficient calories

When you don't consume enough calories, your metabolism may slow down to conserve energy in response to low energy levels. Therefore you end up feeling as though you are not feeling any improvement, irrespective of being on the Keto Diet. In addition, if you create a calorie deficit that is too large, your metabolism rate will drastically drop in order to protect your organs and normal body functions.

You are not eating satiating meals

The Keto Diet is more effective when you stick to it. Eating a super low-calorie meal makes you hungry from time to time. This tends to cause you to deviate from strictly following the Keto Diet. You may even start eating foods that negatively impact ketosis. Often, you find yourself developing cravings for unhealthy foods which alter ketosis. Satiating fats, especially saturated fats and monounsaturated fats, are healthy and provide a great foundation for the Keto Diet. Basically, for the Keto Diet to be successful, you need to identify abundant sources of high quality and healthy fats. For example, MCT oils are the most preferred because they are more satiating than coconut oil. They boost ketone production and can re-ignite ketosis.

You are over-engaging in exercising

Exercising is crucial to improving your overall health. Nevertheless, there is a healthy limit of exercising for everyone. Too much of anything can be bad. Excessive exercising increases your appetite since much fat and many calories are burned. Appetite increases because the body needs a replenishment of the fats and calories depleted during exercising.

You do not get enough sleep

Sleeping is always underestimated as an important factor that facilitates several processes in the body. Inadequate sleep can throw off circadian rhythms and increase the risk of metabolic complications. Sleeping is important in hormonal balancing which facilitates continuous and stable ketosis. For example, satisfying sleep regulates the hunger hormones ghrelin and leptin. Insufficient levels of these hormones cause you to skip meals, which assists ketosis.

You regularly experience stress

Scientists suggest that stress causes a high production of cortisol, a hormone that the body releases when under high pressure or in a panic. The hormone then channels glucose to the muscles.

The hormone increases the storage of fats in the stomach. Cortisol is a problem when its production becomes chronic due to stress. The fat stored in the stomach starts to increase. Generally, the accumulation of fat in the stomach may pose a health problem.

What to Do When Traveling and Eating Out

Occasionally, you may want to go out on a date or any other social situation. Humans are social beings who usually share a meal or drinks as a show of goodwill. It is good to handle any social situation with grace and confidence without anyone noticing you are refraining from some foods. Even when you are on the Keto Diet, you can go out and enjoy a meal with friends, relatives, and colleagues. It will not be a big deal!

However, it is tricky to eat everything on the restaurant menu while on the Keto Diet. Thus, below are a few things you should consider when you are traveling and eating out.

Eat enough before going out

This may sound unrealistic, especially when you know the delicacies available in a restaurant you want to visit. It may appear unfair to restrict yourself while other people are enjoying all sorts of foods. However, do not forget that you on a special diet that includes dietary restrictions.

Therefore, it would be wise to eat a delicious keto meal before you go out or travel. You'll be less concerned about the non-keto delicacies other are enjoying. By eating a light meal before going out or traveling, you are less likely to eat unhealthy foods because of impromptu snacking. Alternatively, you can pack some keto snacks.

Skip the meal

If you are out for lunch or dinner and find no keto foods on the menu, just skip the meal. One meal is not worth undoing your progress. Remind yourself that the Keto Diet only becomes effective when you remain loyal. Persistence and commitment to keto meals will go a long way toward enhancing the impact of the Keto Diet. In short, one junk food meal is not worth to ruin your hard-earned dedication to the Keto Diet.

Stick to the meat dishes

It is true that restaurants may not have prepared keto meals. Nevertheless, almost all restaurants serve steak. It's best to avoid the fries and go just for the meat, which is in line with Keto Diet meals and will enhance ketosis. Pork chops can also serve the same purpose. Getting some chicken breast covered in mozzarella cheese is also a great option. Request that no sauce is added to your meat pieces.

Do not be afraid to ask questions

If you are not sure about the meals served, do not hesitate to ask the waiter questions. The restaurant may have prepared foods that conform to the Keto Diet. If you do not ask and assume that you cannot get keto foods in a restaurant, you may starve yourself for no good reason. Otherwise, you can order a special meal and the chefs will be happy to oblige.

Here are examples of things you can request to be on the

safe side:

- If you are ordering seafood or meat, ensure the waiter knows that you don't want anything breaded.

- Request food that does not contain spices. Tell the waiter to bring a spice shaker if you need some. Do not forget that most spices contain carbs.

- Ask your waiter for salads which contain olive oil or red wine vinegar dressings.

- Do not hesitate to let the waiter know you are sensitive to certain foods. If there is no food that conforms to the Keto Diet, try the next restaurant or food joint.

Order vegetables on the side

Some restaurants prefer providing set options as a side because they are cheaper. Replace them by ordering some sautéed or steamed vegetables dressed with butter. Do not ruin your diet plans because the restaurant doesn't offer appropriate veggies. Choose something else.

Research the restaurant beforehand

It is wise to research the restaurant or hotel you are about to visit. You'll save yourself the frustration of being at a hotel where you cannot find any meal to eat. Visit their website and read through their menu to get important dietary information. This will help you determine whether or not it is worthwhile to go the hotel. Preferably, scrutinize the menu to see whether they serve something with no added sugars or offer any keto foods.

Order a customized meal

Why should you eat foods just because they appear on the menu? You can always order a personalized meal in any restaurant. As crazy as it appears, go on and order some beef steak with veggies and sour cream. It is not bad and will help you stay in ketosis.

Moreover, request that pancake batter not be added to your scrambled eggs and omelets. Let the chef know that you would appreciate it if you got whole fried eggs. Get more meat or chicken than processed meats such as bacon, sausages, and meat pies, among others. They may contain sugar ingredients, spices, and additives that may not be favorable to ketosis.

Avoid Overeating

It is inappropriate to eat more than your stomach can tolerate. Even as you are traveling, or out for lunch or dinner, and you coincidentally find keto food at a restaurant, do not overeat. Restaurants are fond of serving large amounts which are often more than one person should consume. When eating out on the Keto Diet, share the extra portion with a friend. If alone, put a share of the meal in a takeout container before eating.

Keto Meal Plans

There are different types of keto diets. The various categories are discussed below.

Classic Keto

The classic Keto Diet is the original ketogenic diet that was designed for the treatment of epilepsy. Basically, it suggests an intake of fat and proteins and carbs in a 4:1ratio. However, the fat content may be altered for a more therapeutic outcome. The classic Keto Diet is the most conventional way to deal with autism and epilepsy in children.

Full Keto

The full Keto Diet mainly incorporates a higher intake of fats compared to other macros. The majority of dieters on this plan start to experience ketosis within the first one week.

Adapted Fat Burner

By reducing your carb intake, your body switches to using fats as a source of energy. When the process continues for a few weeks, you become an adapted fat burner. At that point, you can eat as much fat as you want without experiencing any side effects. When you become fat adapted, you are able to go for four to six hours without feeling hungry.

Daily Fat Burner

When you become fat adapted, you can consume more than 100grams of fats in one single meal. In this meal plan, one develops the capability for burning an extremely high amount of fat. People who exercise on a daily basis burn even more fat. When you are a daily fat burner, you should align your meals with a lot of fats. While taking on the daily fat burner Keto Diet plan, maximize the intake of quality fats. The more fats you consume in your meals, the better.

Chapter Five

Complete 90-Day Plan 30 Pounds Or More

Losing weight requires proper dieting. **While you can lose weight on a particular diet, exercising is a catalyst. Therefore, note that dietary measures are paramount and should be your first method of losing weight.** Losing 30 pounds can be overwhelming and is for at least 90 days. To make it easier, try and set small and achievable goals. For example, you can aim at losing half a pound of body mass per day. If you find that hard, you can alternatively set a weekly weight loss goal of at least three pounds. Ensure you weigh yourself every week to determine whether or not your routine is being successful. If you are successful for the first time, it means that you should be motivated to set new goals.

This is a complete 90-day plan to lose 30 pounds, divided into two main parts—dietary and exercise measures. It contains a sample meal and workout timetables. Below are the tips to guide you in losing 30 pounds or more.

Dietary Measures That Cause Weight Loss

Knowing What You Eat

Weight loss requires eating more natural foods and avoiding processed foods. This translates to filing your diet with real, whole foods and healthy proteins sources such as poultry, eggs, lean meat, and beans. Also, you can include beneficial carbs such as oatmeal, brown rice, and fruits. Healthy fats and oils sources like avocados, olive oil, and nuts should not be left out.

Avoid foods such as cake, cookies, and other unhealthy foods. Sugary and high-fat foods will only make your efforts to lose weight futile. It is prudent to restructure your meals to ensure that the ingredients are low fat, low calorie, and low sugar. Eat more protein and fiber-rich foods.

Overconsumption of junk and processed foods is one of the worst habits you can have while trying to lose weight. Eating junk food reduces energy levels and increases the risk for myriad diseases, increases blood pressure, increases the likelihood of type 2 diabetes, and much more. Definitely, this will affect the efficiency of your weight loss endeavors.

Choosing a Weight-Loss Diet Plan

A perfect weight loss diet plan should have a practical schedule which is easy to follow. It should indicate what to eat for effective weight loss. Additionally, it should lead to serious impacts on your body such as improved health, better concentration, and overall body mass. There are a number of diet plans deemed to have weight loss effects. It is best to consult a dietician for more advice concerning the diet plan that fits you.

The Keto Diet is one of the best diet plans for weight loss. When you begin consuming keto meals, you are satiated most of the times and can therefore skip some meals. Furthermore, you burn more fat for energy. You will start witnessing changes in your body mass. While on the Keto Diet, you should formulate a timetable for your meals and ensure that you include healthy keto foods. Below is an example of a timetable for a weight loss Keto Diet.

Day Meal	Monday	Tuesday	Wednesday
Breakfast	An omelet served with cheese and veggies. Mushrooms, cooked in coconut oil, can	A smoothie with low glucose powder, spinach leaves, avocado, and almond butter. A little milk can be	Boiled eggs with sautéed greens such as spinach

	also do.	added.	
Lunch	Blueberries and cottage cheese	Tuna salad lettuce wraps with pork	Grilled chicken or bacon with lettuce or salad. Avocado chunks can be eaten too.
Dinner	Zucchini with crispy baked salmon	Slow-cooked beef cooked with shredded cabbage. Cooked with red onions, soy sauce, butter, garlic and red pepper flakes	Olive oil, cream, butter, and roasted zucchini with baked salmon and cauliflower
Thursday	**Friday**	**Saturday**	**Sunday**
Intermittent Fasting Day (Breakfast at 8 a.m.) 2or 3 fried eggs and bacon	Plain Greek yogurt with a spoonful of almond butter	Ribs and zucchini, cooked with coconut oil for better taste	2 or 3 fried eggs and bacon with a glass of a smoothie
(Lunch at 11 a.m.) Grilled chicken breast with about six cherry tomatoes	Grilled chicken breast with lettuce and avocado dressing	Mexican chicken wrapped up with lettuce and a whole avocado	Spinach salad with fried lean meat
(Dinner at 2 p.m.)	Rice cooked in olive oil with beef and	Tortilla (Tacos)	Roasted pork rubbed with sea salt and

beef steak with a glass of coconut milk (20-30 mins after eating)	broccoli or cauliflower. Butter and other fat add-ons like cheese can be added to enhance the taste		garlic. Cauliflower with mashed potatoes made with heavy cream, butter, and olive oil can be added.

Note: You can include your own choice of snack. During the intermittent fasting day, you should not have a snack.

The best diet plan should provide a tool for monitoring your progress. You should be motivated to continue to lose a significant weight in the course of the three months.

Intermittent Fasting

Based on various studies conducted to establish the best ways to enhance weight loss, intermittent fasting is a viable and healthy method. Intermittent fasting involves eating only in a specified time frame. Basically, it entails allocating a strict eating period to a section of a day. For example, one can choose to eat only between 8:00 a.m. and 2:00 p.m. (six hours). This eating method enhances weight loss by limiting the amount of food you consume in a day.

When you reduce the amount of food consumed, the

amount of glucose in the body is also reduced. Consequently, the body begins to look for another source of energy. The only other available source of energy in the body is body fat. The liver starts breaking down the fat into energy. In the process, a lot of body fat is converted into energy. Burning body fat means reducing body mass, which leads to weight loss.

Exercise That Enhances Weight Loss

As indicated above, exercising should not be the first option in the process of losing weight. It just enhances how fast you lose weight.

Do More Cardiovascular Exercise

Start a cardiovascular training plan that will enhance how your body burns calories and increases your metabolisms. According to weight loss experts, cardio workouts are vital for helping anyone to lose weight. These workouts may include biking, jogging, swimming, aerobics, dancing, skiing, sprinting, and walking. If quick weight loss is desired, one should aim at doing cardio exercises for no less than five days a week. Otherwise, the workouts can be alternated throughout the week. That means one cardio workout for every week. To be effective in weight loss, aim for at least 45 to 60 minutes of cardio exercises.

Take up strength training for weight loss

Engaging in strength training exercises has proven to be an effective way to burn quite a lot of calories. The best type of strength training for weight loss is circuit training. Circuit training involves working on major muscles at once. This means that one performs exercises impacting every group of muscles in the body simultaneously. As a result, your body will get toned and sculpted and lead to weight loss. Since the aim is to lose not less than 30 pounds in three months, you can try strength training for six days a week. You should work on your chest, arms, shoulder, back, and abs one day, and your hamstrings, quadriceps, buttocks, and calves the following day.

Endurance training

Any type of training may be a key contributor to weight loss. Likewise, the intensity of endurance training leads to fast weight loss. Ideally, endurance training aims at making the body tolerate long exercising periods but with small break intervals. Endurance training improves the way our bodies burn calories. Research has shown that people who practice endurance training are more likely to lose weight than those who do normal training. Endurance training enhances strength and leads to a healthier body. In addition, muscles grow bigger and the cardiovascular system becomes efficient. Most body parts adapt to functioning effectively and for longer hours.

Below is a workout schedule to give you an idea about what you can do to fast track the 90-day challenge of losing more than 30 pounds. Remember, this is not a requirement, you can lose weight without ever going to the gym!

Period	Monday	Tuesday	Wednesday
Morning	Strength training for the chest and back	1-hour biking cardio exercise	Endurance training (several rounds on a pitch)
Evening	Cardio exercise (swimming)	Strength training arms and shoulders	Cardio exercise (dancing/yoga)

Thursday	Friday	Saturday	Sunday
Rest day	Rest day	Cardio exercise(aerobics)	Endurance training (2 hours of weightlifting)
		Strength training for legs, quadriceps, and buttocks	Cardio exercise(jogging)

Note: The rest days are important for muscle recovery and should never be left out of a training schedule. It should be ample of time to facilitate full muscle recovery.

Chapter Six: FAQs About

The Keto Diet

This section aims to answer the commonly asked questions about the Keto Diet. If you have any other questions, look for more information online. Furthermore, ask your physician or nutritionist to clarify any doubts.

What is the ketogenic (keto) diet?

The Keto Diet is an eating plan that recommends a reduction of carbohydrates in favor of a higher fat intake. The Keto Diet aims to replace sugars with fats as a source of energy in the body.

What are the health benefits of the ketogenic diet?

The health benefits of the Keto Diet are vast. Some benefits include:

- Improved cardiovascular function

- Reduced risk of various diseases like heart

disease

- Enhanced cognitive function

- Weight loss

- Decreased inflammation and oxidative stress

- Stabilized and healthier blood sugar and blood lipid balance

How many carbs should I eat on the ketogenic diet?

Well, the Keto Diet is very clear that one should eat as few carbs as possible. The best answer for this question is that the viable limits for carbs should be between 30 to 100 grams per day. Eating more than 100 grams per day will affect ketosis.

Do I have to count calories or track macros intake on every Keto meal?

If you are sure that what you are eating is keto friendly, there is no need to track your macros. In short, you should not concern yourself with tracking macros if you are eating all foods listed as keto foods. However, you are supposed to track macros if you want to stray from keto foods for a snack or for one meal.

What supplements should I use on the Keto Diet?

Even as the Keto diet may be self-sufficient in providing the body with the required nutrients, supplements can be taken to boost certain deficiencies. However, supplements should be taken with prior consultation and approval of a dietician. Note that an abnormal intake of some supplements can cause enormous effects on the body.

Is cutting out carbs unhealthy for me? Aren't carbohydrates necessary for my body?

Scientifically, your body can survive without consuming any dietary carbohydrates. Therefore, it is not unhealthy to forgo carbs and instead eat more fat with some protein. These two macros can healthily substitute for carbs. Remember that the main use of carbs in the body is energy production, which can be replaced by ketosis (use of fats for energy production).

Is ketosis a dangerous condition for the body?

You must have heard that ketosis is dangerous, especially to keto beginners. Well, it is not dangerous! One may just develop minor systems caused by the keto flu as the body becomes adapted to the Keto Diet. For some people, the flu is usually gone by the end of the first week. However, if the flu prolongs, it cannot go for more than three weeks.

Are there any side effects of cutting out carbs?

Some people experience short-lived irritability, frequent urination, dehydration, and the keto flu. After a short period, the body gets used to a low-carb and high-fat intake.

Why does one feel tired and weak while starting the Keto Diet?

It is because your body metabolism is experiencing dietary changes. Nothing serious though! You just have to be patient for some time (not more than two weeks). Additionally, you can take some energy supplements such as MCT oils and exogenous ketones.

Should I halt alcohol intake behavior while on the Keto Diet?

No! The only thing you should do is reduce your alcohol intake and know the type of alcohol to consume. Do not forget that most alcoholic drinks are very rich in carbs and unfriendly to the Keto Diet. The best option for you is pure spirits in moderate quantities. In addition, do not

mix spirits with soda or fruit juices because the net effect
will be adding to your carb intake.

Is the Keto Diet good for everyone?

No. The Keto Diet is not for everyone. It is generally
better for people who want to lose weight, improve
cognitive function, reduce risks of certain diseases, and
enhance endurance, among other personal goals. If you
don't have any such goals, why bother with keto?

How is loss weight achieved on the Keto Diet?

This is probably the most common question among
people who want to start the Keto Diet. The Keto Diet
leads to burning of body fat to produce energy. Ideally,
this will lead to weight loss.

Do I need to regularly track ketone levels in the body?

It is good to frequently measure the ketone levels in the
body. It will help you fully understand how to regulate
your fat intake. Measuring ketones should go hand in
hand with tracking macros.

What is keto adaptation?

Keto adaptation happens when the body starts shifting away from glucose to fat metabolism. In simple words, it is the process by which the body starts using fat as a source of energy. Keto adaptation occurs in the body tissues such as brains, liver, kidney, and muscles.

Is the Keto Diet suitable for kids?

Yes. The genesis of the Keto Diet was curbing autism and epilepsy in children. This is a clear indication that it is safe for children. It can go a long way in reducing the risk of children developing adverse health complications that are prevalent for youngsters.

Can I use the Keto Diet during pregnancy or while breastfeeding?

The Keto Diet is not safe for expectant and breastfeeding mothers. In fact, the major downside of the diet during these two periods may be weight loss. Losing weight during pregnancy and breastfeeding may have a huge negative impact because fat cells may release toxins. This may have serious effects on the fetus or a nursing baby.

Can vegetarians go keto?

Definitely, yes! It is possible to be a vegetarian and do the Keto Diet. All you need to do is select the most suitable food substitutes for meat. It is relatively easy to combine a vegetarian and Keto Diet.

Can I eat too much fat while on the Keto Diet?

Yes. But too much does not mean excess. "Sufficient" fats should be the ideal word to quantify the levels of fats to be consumed while on keto. Enough fats on the Keto Diet solve caloric deficits. However, do not forget that excess fat will lead to dragon breath and fruity-scented urine and sweat.

Does the Keto Diet have any effect on the kidneys?

Many people are misled by the notion that the Keto Diet may be harmful to the kidneys due to the macro composition. However, the Keto Diet is safe and healthy for the kidneys. More fats in the body do not mean any harm to the kidneys. In fact, the Keto Diet may even be protective to your kidneys, especially if you have diabetes.

I have chronic insulin resistance (type 2 diabetes). Is the Keto Diet safe for me?

Consider getting medical advice first. However, reducing carb intake enhances your body's ability to metabolize insulin. In turn, this helps stabilize blood glucose levels.

Is it true that I should not eat whole eggs because they have a lot of cholesterol?

Eggs are the best-known source of healthy fats in the Keto Diet. There is no conclusive evidence that whole eggs increase LDL cholesterol. In fact, there is research that points to good cholesterol from eggs. Therefore, there is no danger in eating eggs while on the Keto Diet.

Does the Keto Diet increase cholesterol levels since it entails consumption of high volumes of fats?

Actually, research suggests the opposite. Cutting out carbs and focusing on a high-fat intake improves your cholesterol and blood lipid levels. Once the body is in ketosis, it breaks down most fats in the body into ketones to create energy. This ensures that most fats are burned to form energy, reducing the chances of developing high cholesterol levels. Also, it is important to note that fats consumed do not increase triglycerides and lipoproteins in your body.

Are artificial sweeteners allowed on the Keto Diet?

No! Artificial sweeteners can disrupt ketosis. Therefore, it is advisable to avoid them altogether. There are natural sweeteners that can be used in place of artificial sweeteners. For example, stevia is a better option.

Is it possible to lose muscle mass when carbs are cut out of a diet?

Your muscles will not go anywhere as long as you consume sufficient protein and calories. Do not buy into the myth that reducing carbs will diminish your muscles.

I am aiming to build more muscles and increase athletic ability. Is the Keto Diet good for that?

Generally, the Keto Diet can be useful for athletes and bodybuilders. The Keto Diet is a perfect meal which supplies enough ketones (energy) to muscles. In turn, training endurance is boosted and bodybuilding becomes easy. In fact, most endurance athletes find the Keto Diet is a beneficial long-term source of energy. This is because macros combination in the Keto Diet is great in enhancing aerobic and cardiovascular stamina.

Does the low-carb diet in keto make urine smell fruity?

Yes. This is attributed to the natural scent of ketones that are excreted in the urine. It is not something to be worried about. Furthermore, it is only for a short time (a maximum of two weeks).

Does being on keto mean that you are not supposed to eat sugary foods?

Surprisingly, the first few weeks of the Keto Diet are the only period you should be strict about limiting your sugar intake. Afterward, you can eat sugary foods but only in moderate amounts. You have to ensure that you limit the levels of carbs in every meal to enhance ketosis.

What should I do when I develop cravings for sugary foods while on Keto?

It would be prudent to forfeit your cravings for sugary foods while on the Keto Diet. Alternatively, opt for any of the sweeteners listed in this book as keto friendly. Many people only have sugar craving during the first few days of keto. When the body gets used to the Keto Diet, you will have a craving for fatty foods like nuts, cheese, and meat.

How much water should I drink while on the Keto Diet?

Water is important regardless of whether or not you are on the Keto Diet. You should drink eight to 12 glasses of water daily. During the first few days of keto, you should drink up to 12 glasses or more to replenish water lost through frequent urination.

What does being in ketosis mean?

Being in ketosis simply means that your liver is producing ketones to supply the body with energy. While you are in ketosis, your body has already started using ketones as its only source of energy. Glucose is no longer the source of energy for your body.

What may put me out of ketosis and how can I get back into it quickly?

Mainly, ketosis is lowered by not consuming enough fats. Additionally, you lower ketosis whenever you increase your intake of carbs. You can get back into ketosis by consuming the recommended amounts of fats while abstaining from carbs. Furthermore, you can incorporate periods of fasting combined with keto fats such as MTCs.

How often will I feel hungry while on the Keto Diet?

One of the most surprising things about the Keto Diet is that you always feel full. While you go keto, hunger pangs between meals begin to fade away. You remain satiated for a longer period than when you are on normal meals. This is why people use the Keto Diet to lose weight, since you rarely feel the need to eat.

Are there any simple recipes for tasty keto meals?

Of course! There are numerous sources of Keto Diet recipes. The majority of them are websites, eBooks, and magazines. The appendix of this eBook lists some websites where keto recipes can be found.

What is the lowest body fat percentage that is healthy?

According to many dieticians, the essential body fat should be eight to twelve percent for women and three to five percent for men. A dieter should not go below this level for effective Keto diet plan.

Is Ketosis safe for diabetics?

The Keto Diet automatically leads to Ketosis which is generally very powerful treatment in reversing type 2 diabetes. Additionally, patients with type 1 diabetes can employ the Keto diet in improving their blood sugar control. However, insulin injections should continue as usual but on lower doses. All this should be done with the consultation of a doctor. Generally, patients of both type 1 and type 2 diabetes require a reduction of medication on the Keto diet to avoid hypoglycemia.

How many carbs can you eat and still be in Ketosis?

The ideal amount of carbs to take while on the Keto Diet is above 20 grams per days. However, it is imperative to note that people who are not insulin resistant can sometimes tolerate more carbs. For this reason, they may have almost 50 grams of carbs per day.

Can I have fruits on a Keto Diet?

Fruits are healthy. However, most of them contain very high amounts of carbs and sugars which may not favor Ketosis. Therefore, when it comes to fruits, choose most of the fruits indicated in the grocery list or those that your dietician may recommend for the Keto Diet.

What's the difference between low-carb and Keto Diets?

The main difference is in the volume of carbs that each plan advocate. Keto Diet is strict than a low carb diet. In fact, a low carb diet does not specify the quantity of carbs to be taken. The Keto Diet plan is clear on the percentage of carbs that should be included in a meal. Thus, the Keto could be called an extra strict low-carb diet.

At what time of the day should you test Ketone levels?

Measuring Ketones in the morning before eating anything is the best practice. This will give a dieter a clear comparison of the Ketone levels throughout the day. It also makes it easier to compare Ketone levels from day to day. Dieters should note Ketones are low in the morning and higher in the evening.

What is fat fasting?

Basically, fat fasting is a type of fasting where a dieter eats about 90 percent of calorie from fat. Carbs are forfeited while fats are consumed in line with the outlined amounts.

My friend is on Keto and often soak nuts and seeds. Is this a good practice and why?

Soaked nuts are known to have more health benefits than raw nuts. Before roasting, one can soak the nuts. This is because they are better digested and their nutrients are better absorbed. Soaking helps in reducing phytic acids present in the nuts and seeds.

Are peanuts healthy for the Keto Diet?

Like other legumes, peanuts still remain a controversial food among people who follow the Keto diet. Peanuts are known to contain anti-nutrients that can reduce their nutritional value and cause health issues in vulnerable individuals. However, they are low carb legumes and this makes them Keto friendly.

Does the Keto Diet cause vitamin and mineral deficiency?

The loss of certain minerals and vitamins during Ketosis is a major risk concern associated with the Keto Diet. However, this is not a permanent situation since one can reverse the loss of these minerals by taking specific foods. The foods should be rich in the minerals and vitamins in question. Moreover, dieters may take supplements but with the guidance of a dietician.

Can the Keto Diet improve acid reflux?

According to studies, yes it can! People living with the discomfort and reduced quality of life from acid reflux exhibit positive results while under the Keto Diet.

Will I lose muscle mass if I cut out carbs?

No! As long as you consume enough proteins and calories, your muscle tissues will remain intact. Actually, sufficient intake of the two combined with some exercise will build your muscles bigger and stronger.

Is there a better way to cycle Keto Dieting?

Since coping and managing the strict Keto diet is hard for almost every dieter, there is a chance for a healthy change. One common alternative is using the Keto Diet for a short period throughout the year with a conservative bridge between Keto Diet and normal carb dieting.

Can type I diabetics follow the Keto Diet?

As mentioned earlier, any diabetic patient is free to follow the Keto diet. However, there must be close medical supervision. This is because type 1 diabetics may get into a dangerous Ketoacidosis if not closely monitored by an expert.

Is the Keto Diet suitable for women going through menopause?

Yes! There are no validated negative effects of the Keto Diet to women going through menopause. Generally, we cannot attribute the Keto Diet to any health complications that women may experience during menopause.

APPENDIX

Where to Get More Info and Keto Recipes

Many people ask where they can get keto recipes and more information about the Keto Diet. Below are the most preferred websites which provide comprehensive recipes for snacks, breakfast, lunch, and dinner.

- https://ketodietapp.com

- https://www.ruled.me

- https://ketosummit.com

- https://www.ketovangelist.com

- https://rw.yourketo.diet

- https://www.dietdoctor.com

- https://www.perfectketo.com

- https://ketosizeme.com

- https://lowcarbyum.com

- https://ketogasm.com

- https://low-carb-support.com

- https://thedailynutrition.com

- https://ketologic.com

- https://www.ketodomain.com

- https://ketodash.com

- https://bioketo.com

Thank You!

Before you go, we would like to thank you for purchasing a copy of our book. Out of the dozens of books you could have picked over ours, you decided to go with this one and for that we are very grateful.

We hope you enjoyed reading it as much as we enjoyed writing it! We hope you found it very informative.

We would like to ask you for a small favor. <u>Could you please take a moment to leave a review for this book on Amazon?</u>

Your feedback will help us continue to write more books and release new content in the future!

Made in the USA
Columbia, SC
16 August 2018